Ayurvedic Medicine for Westerners

Volume 1

Anatomy and Physiology in Ayurveda

Vaidya Atreya Smith

Other books by Vaidya Atreya Smith:

Prana the Secret of Yogic Healing, Samuel Weiser, 1996

Practical Ayurveda, Samuel Weiser, 1998

Ayurvedic Healing for Women, Samuel Weiser, 1999

Secrets of Ayurvedic Massage, Lotus Press, 2000

Perfect Balance, Avery Publishing, 2001

Ayurvedic Nutrition Course Textbook, Editions Turiya, 2001

Pañcakarma - Shodhana Chikitsā Textbook, Editions Turiya, 2003

Ayurvedic Nutrition, CreateSpace, 2010

The Psychology of Transformation in Yoga, CreateSpace, 2013

Ayurvedic Medicine for Westerners, Vol. 3; Dravyaguna for Westerners, 2013

www.atreya.com

ISBN-13: 978-1491043905

ISBN-10: 1491043903

DEDICATION

This textbook is dedicated to my students.

CONTENTS

ACKNOWLEDGMENTS

I would like to acknowledge the many teachers I have had and continue to have in India. With their guidance Ayurveda is growing the West. I also wish to thank the many patients I have seen over the last twenty-five years that have made Ayurveda come alive for me in clinical practice.

INTRODUCTION

This textbook on Ayurveda came into being over the last nineteen years. As a practitioner since 1987 and teacher of Ayurveda since 1994 I have used a variety of sources and material to teach from over the years. Everything from Indian classics to books by Western authors of Ayurveda have passed through my hands over the years. As with most professionals in any domain we tend to prefer our own work, views, ideas and concepts – especially when teaching.

Thus, this series of textbooks that I am presenting now in book form are simply the accumulation of written material I have used to teach lessons to my students over the last nineteen years. Most of Ayurveda is classic and does not change much from textbook to textbook. There are, however, small details that each author brings to every subject that can be of great benefit to the struggling student. Therefore, another textbook is not 'out of line' in the greater scheme of things. Additionally, each teacher has a different view of things and manner of expressing these views which can be helpful.

There are several points that have irritated me as a teacher over the years (which is one reason why I began to write my own lessons) that I feel obliged to point out to the new or intermediate student. The main issues I have are:

1. Non practitioners writing medical texts
2. Mixing personal ideas or opinions with classical knowledge
3. The blending of esoteric, new-age, magic or pseudo-spirituality in textbooks

The first point was a great deception for me personally. As a practitioner first and foremost I was often at a loss to understand why information in some textbooks, course books or general books on Ayurveda would not work with my patients in Europe. I found out quickly that what I had learned in India during the six years of residency there from 1987 to the end of 1994 needed to be adapted to a different climate, culture, food, herbs and psychology. The other aspect of my failure to get results took me much longer to discover. The main problem was that most of the books or manuals I was using were written by non-medical and non-practicing authors. In essence much of what is written about Ayurveda in therapeutic applications simply does not work because it is wrong, or has never been tested in clinical environments.

This is, of course, true in any system of medicine. There has always been and probably always will be the scholars, researchers of medicine and the practitioners of medicine. When the two of these camps meet we often get valuable insights and information on the given subject. This is one of my primary goals: to write a textbook on Ayurveda for Western people that is based on practical clinical experience. To what extent I will be able to achieve this goal will only be known with time.

This will explain to Indian doctors and students why many classical sections of information may be missing from this series of textbooks. As I am basically a practitioner and not a scholar of Ayurveda I am presenting only the aspects of Ayurveda that I have personally found important in the practice of Ayurveda in Europe. Obviously this is subjective and some aspects of Ayurveda that are important to Indians practicing in India may be missing. However, the goal of this series of books is to bring a practical textbook on Ayurveda to the serious Western practitioner of Ayurveda, not to add to the already abundant literature that already exists in India.

The second issue I have is with authors and teachers who mix their personal ideas and experiences in with classical information on Ayurveda. Basically this is deceiving the student. For the teacher to tread the path of Dharma, or correct conduct, it is highly important to indicate to the student the classical information, the information from modern authors, and finally, their own experience of what works. Given this opportunity the student can approach the clinical experience of Ayurveda with an open mind and try to see what works and what doesn't. Too often I run into students who say, "Dr. So and So says this so it is like this". Or worse, "There are 100 trillion Agni in the body because that is what I learned from Dr. So and So". Certainly, one can argue that the human body has 100 trillion cells, and each of these cells has Agni within it. Nothing wrong with stating your opinion. Unfortunately, for the trusting student the classics state there are thirteen forms of Agni, not 100 trillion. The failure of the teacher to clarify what is classical or their opinion is at the very least a disservice to the serious student.

The *Caraka Samhita* (considered by most scholars to be the oldest text on Ayurveda) is basically a dialog of teachers and students discussing Ayurveda, social issues and life in general. Ayurveda is a body of knowledge that is open and changes according to the vision or approach. It is most certainly not a fixed vision of health care or life. It has also changed historically according to different societies and cultures. Thus, teachers that try to dictate to their students the "finality" of any subject are distorting Ayurveda and handicapping their students for further study. Often this rebounds on the teacher as the student becomes disillusioned by the miss-information at a later date.

The third issue I have with books and textbooks on Ayurveda is the ego promoting use of so called 'esoteric knowledge' mixed in with classical Ayurveda. Worse still is the pseudo-spiritual lines of the self-promoting author or teacher. Ayurveda has a rich spiritual tradition and has a variety of spiritual paths that it encompasses. It is not necessary for self-proclaimed gurus to add in worthless information that confuses the serious student.

Stories abound around the teacher who tells of miracle cures. The real *Vaidya* – knower of Ayurveda – is able to take whatever substances are in the kitchen or garden and use them to reduce the suffering of the patient. Yes, of course, we would all love a fully stocked clinic with magical cows urine and hundred year old ghee; unfortunately this is not Ayurveda. Ayurvedic medicine is a codified system of knowledge that allows the practitioner to understand the patient and find anything from nature (under any circumstances) that will restore proper homeostasis. Ayurveda is not about mysterious yogis in the Himalayas that transmit special forms of diagnosis to the worthy doctor – and of course the humble doctor who received this information will let you know how humble and worthy he is!

Ayurveda already has a rich spiritual tradition as it is an *Upaveda* or one of the classical branches of Vedic knowledge. The Indian tradition is rich in mystery and it is best if the serious student discovers these mysteries on their own and not with the 'help' of self-promoting teachers. The worst aspect of this from my point of view is that the student stops investigating therapeutic options. They are told that, "only the secret mantra from my dead teacher will cure this disease" and other such cow dung. Being taught in this manner is not along the Vedic tradition. The Vedic tradition encourages creative discussion and thinking among students, not magical mantras or medicines.

Having said my peace I will now let the students decide if this series of textbooks has any merit or not. I have received help from many quarters over the last twenty-five years of practicing Ayurveda and I wish most of all to thank my many patients (who most likely will never read this) for bringing an enormous variety of disorders and diseases to me. Thanks to the Blessings of the Ayurveda I hope that I have helped most of them.

Vaidya Atreya Smith
December 2013

CHAPTER ONE
SAMKHYA DARSHANA

It is not possible to begin the study of Ayurveda without having the social and philosophical context of the system explained or reviewed. The Vedic seers who codified Ayurveda over centuries "saw" the world in a specific manner. This seeing is called *Darshana* in Sanskrit and literally means "to see". In order to understand the context of how Ayurveda is visualized in India we need to keep an open mind to their cultures' basic precept that everything occurring in the creation is alive with an intelligent consciousness. The idea is that 'Darshana' is a verb – indicating the action and movement of *seeing* – this is very important to correctly understand Ayurvedic medicine. The 'seeing' action associated with all Darshana means that reality can be observed and studied. These are the *Shaddarshanas* or the six systems of Indian "philosophy":

1. Nyaya Darshana
2. Vaisesika Darshana
3. Samkhya Darshana
4. Yoga Darshana
5. Purva Mimamsa Darshana
6. Uttara Mimamsa or Vedanta Darshana

They generally deal with four topics:

1. Existence and nature of *Brahman* / Pure Consciousness / God
2. Nature of the *jiva* / *jivatman* or the individual soul
3. Creation of the *jagat* or the material world
4. *Moksha* / liberation or enlightenment and the disciplines that lead to it

Briefly they can be described as follows:

1.   Nyaya Darshana - Traditionally founded by *Akshapada Gautama* (6th cent. B.C.), is a school of logic and epistemology that defined the rules of debate, the canons of proof and accepted means of acquiring knowledge. Its views are accepted with minor modifications by the other schools.

2.   Vaisesika Darshana - The atomist school founded by *Kanada* (3d cent. B.C.), analyzed reality into six categories: substance, quality, activity, generality, particularity, and

inherence. The universe is made up of nine kinds of substance: earth, water, light, air, ether, time, space, soul (*jivatman*), and mind. Pure Consciousness (God) is regarded as the fundamental force who causes consciousness in these atoms by His Divine will.

3.   Samkhya Darshana - Traditionally expounded by *Kapila* (6th cent. B.C.), is based on two basic metaphysical principles, *Purusha* (Pure Consciousness) and *Prakriti* (Latent Matter) and is generally considered to dualistic in nature. Prakriti consists of three Gunas or qualities: *Sattva, Rajas,* and *Tamas.* Disturbance of Prakriti by Purusha initiates a process of creation that ultimately produces both the material world and individual faculties of the human being. Samkhya is regarded as the oldest of the orthodox systems in Vedic thought and existed before Rishi Kapila codified it as a system. There are different interpretations that are non-dualistic such as from the Yoga and Vedanta Darshanas.

4.   Yoga Darshana - Traditionally expounded by *Patanjali* (2d cent. B.C.) accepts Samkhya metaphysics to explain the validity of yogic processes described in the Yoga Sutras and also accepts the concept of an *Ishvara,* individualized or personal God. Yoga is defined as "cessation of the modifications of consciousness" and is achieved by an eight-stage discipline called *astangayoga.* The Samkhya gives primary importance to *tattwajnana* or enquiry into the nature of truth while the Yoga deals primarily with *sadhanas* or spiritual disciplines to attain *Moksha.*

5.   Purva Mimamsa Darshana - The Purva (earlier) Mimamsa school is traditionally founded by *Jaimini* (2d cent. B.C.), and set forth sophisticated principles for interpreting the Veda. This basis is primarily composed of injunctions to ritualistic action. Its epistemology and theory of meaning were constructed to show that the words of the Veda had eternal and intrinsic validity. It forms the basis of Hindu ritualistic practices and *pujas.*

6.   Uttara Mimamsa or Vedanta Darshana - The Uttara (later) Mimamsa school commonly known as *Vedanta,* concentrates on the philosophical teachings of the *Upanishads* rather than on the ritualistic injunctions of the *Brahmanas;* both of which are part of the four Vedas. Vedanta is a form of *Jnana Yoga* out of the four basic yoga practices, the other three Yoga's being, *Raja Yoga, Bhakti Yoga* and *Karma Yoga.* It deals with the individual who seeks the path of discrimination of truth from the untruth. For some scholars it encompasses all the four yoga's. *Rishi Badarayana* is the proponent of this Darshana and the author of the *Brahma Sutras* which are based on the Upanishads.

The first two Darshanas are often classified as being "materialistic" because they deal with logic, the right methods of gaining knowledge, the physical universe, etc. This is not really correct as logic is also used to prove the existence of a divine principle. The atomic vision is also based on the creation beginning from divine will or a Pure Consciousness. Most of these Darshana are attributed to one sage of Rishi which is not really correct. Each view of creation is referred to in some way in the Vedas and is part of Vedic thinking. The Rishi that is attributed to the vision is the last one to codify it into its present form; this is especially true for the Samkhya, Yoga and Vedanta Darshanas.

All of the six Darshana accept that reality can be observed and studied. Hence, there is an intelligent, conscious principle that is able to carry out this observation. The primary basis of these Darshana is that there is a Pure Consciousness that permeates the universe. Whether or not we accept this concept is immaterial. What is important is that Ayurvedic medicine is based on the infallible knowledge that nature is conscious intelligence in action. This intelligence encases itself deeper and deeper into matter as the manifestation of matter occurs. Ayurvedic anatomy and physiology reflect this intelligence. Trying to approach Ayurveda without this understanding leads to numerous and profound misunderstandings. Hence, the study of this physical science should begin with the study of how the body manifests in the first place.

Ayurvedic medicine uses all six of the Darshanas to some extent, but mainly the first three: Nyaya, Vaisesika, Samkhya. Of these three the Samkhya is main vision of creation used. The Samkhya is the oldest and most used of all six Darshana in Vedic thought and Ayurveda is no exception. Samkhya brings a number of important concepts that are fundament to the correct use of Ayurveda as a medical system.

The Samkhya system has several main components, they are in order:

Purusha	0	latent
Prakriti	1	causal
Mahat	1	internal
Ahamkara	1	internal
Manas	1	internal
Tanmatra	5	subtle
Panchamahabuhta	5	external
Jnanendriya	5	external
Karmendriya	5	external

The Samkhya is considered to a logical progression of Pure Consciousness (Purusha) into Latent matter (Prakriti) that gives birth to the creation. Classical Samkhya lists one causal Tattva, three internal Tattvas, five subtle Tattvas and fifteen external Tattvas (see above). A *Tattva* is an element or aspect of reality, the Samkhya Darshana has twenty-four Tattvas. Purusha as Pure Consciousness is not considered to be a Tattva, rather it is latent in all of the following Tattvas. Before defining these terms it is best to try and understand what is the 'system of enumeration' or Samkhya Darshana that forms the basis of Ayurveda? First of all Samkhya is not a philosophy, which presents the primary problem in using or studying the system. There is no actual term that can be used to explain what the Samkhya exactly is – hence, the common translation of 'system of enumeration' or the order of manifestation. This meaning is close to the actual Sanskrit word Samkhya. A loose translation of Samkhya Darshana could be: "The observation and experience of manifestation in a logical, linear and progressive manner, on all levels, in the entire universe, known or unknown to promote the experience of consciousness."

For lack of any better term modern scholars in both the East and West have attached the word 'philosophy' to the Samkhya vision of manifestation. In simple language the Samkhya vision shows us how Pure Consciousness is the origin of all creation and stays within the created manifestation all through the process of creation. Thus, all creation has a fragment of this Pure Consciousness and is therefore conscious. The Samkhya also shows us that the creation is a continual process – it is not fixed in time; and it can be observed.

It also means that everything in creation is in perpetual movement and therefore not static or fixed; indicated further by the use of the verb *Darshana*. Hence, Ayurvedic medicine is also based on the concept that everything in creation is in movement. As a medical system Ayurveda puts the main emphasis on the constant movement of the creation. This movement is linier and defined by the word 'Samkhya' which indicates a clear progression in the manifestation. These concepts are especially important in pathology and treatment modules.

Therefore, Ayurveda is a medical system that is based on the following facts:

1. That the physical universe is observable
2. That the physical universe is in constant movement
3. That the physical universe is in constant change
4. That there is a linear progression to the manifestation of the physical universe
5. And lastly that all of the above are interrelated and in constant interaction

The result of these five points is that Ayurveda is a *functional* system of medicine that is concerned by the *interrelation* and *interaction* of *observable* systems and structures that are in constant *movement* and *change*. In other words because of the Samkhya Darshana Ayurveda is not a static system; by its very nature it is in a system based on change and therefore more concerned with function than with structure.

Purusha – Latent Consciousness

From the unknowable substratum arises *Purusha* or 'pure consciousness'. The *Upanishads*, ancient scriptures of Vedic India, have several names for the substratum. Some of these are: *Paratman, Parabrahman* or Self. It is not possible to give more information the "substratum" because it is prior to consciousness itself. Some people wrongly interpret the Samkhya system as being a dualistic vision of life and creation – it is not. Purusha is a monistic principle and has no concept of dualism inherent within it. Purusha arises from the substratum for no reason. It is hard for the conceptual mind to accept that there can be an event or action without any reason. Nevertheless, this is a very fundamental point of the Vedas, Upanishads and Samkhya Darshana – there is no reason behind the creation. For example see Brhadāranyaka Upanishad, chapter one and the commentary of Shankarācarya

"Some say that creation is for the enjoyment of Purusha, while others say it is only for His indulgence. Actually creation is the nature of Purusha for what desire can He have whose desires are always fulfilled?"
Māndūkya Upanishad, āgama-prakarana, 1.9

Samkhya begins with the Purusha – pure consciousness in a latent or un-manifested state. Purusha is sometimes called *Atman* or *Brahman* in texts. Most people are not able to make a clear distinction between Purusha and the indescribable, unknowable substratum. Purusha is not possible to 'know' either, but it has been given three qualities that are used to help understand it. Unlike the substratum (where there is no possibility to give it any quality - *nirguna*) Purusha, pure consciousness, can be given three primary qualities. Even though Purusha is impossible to define and unknowable we are given the means to recognize it through its three attributes – *Satcitanand*, or Sat (Beingness), Chit (Consciousness), and Ananda (Blissfulness).

Purusha cannot be talked about simply because it is not possible to describe it beyond sat, chit, ananda (Being, Consciousness, Bliss). All of the *Rishi's* (seers) of the past have failed to describe it directly – many have become poets in some attempt to describe it. Others have chosen to remain silent as they saw the futility of trying to describe the indescribable. The only way to comprehend Purusha is to become It. In the attempt to intellectualize Purusha we miss it. It is enough to know that it is latent, un-manifested or existing as a pure potential. To try and go beyond that is to miss the point.

One other classical definition from the Upanishads and Samkhya is that Purusha is eternal – it has no beginning or end (for example see Brhadāranyaka Upanishad, 1.iv.1 to 1.iv.5 and the commentary of Shankarācarya and Rig-Veda, X.129.1-4). In some schools of Samkhya this is used to define what is reality. The logic is that if something manifests and then un-manifests it is not real. By this definition the human body is not real because it is born, grows and dies. Because of this there are several schools that declare the world to be "non-reality" or "illusion" (*Maya*). However, to take this literally misses the point of the original observation.

The emphasis is on the eternal nature of Purusha – pure consciousness – not the transient nature of the manifestation. People wrongly put the emphasis on the manifestation and declare that "everything is illusion" using this to justify unloving behavior towards their family, friends, ignore social responsibilities, or simply to justify general selfish behavior. At the very least it causes mental deception. The school of "all is illusion" is valid provided the student understands the meaning and purpose of the teaching. That teaching is to confirm that only Purusha, that which is unchanging consciousness, is real. Why? Because it is always there, never changing and everything else arises out of it.

Another aspect of this same observation is that of "everything is consciousness". All things arise from Purusha as we shall see, hence, as pure consciousness is the source of all the manifestation everything can be said to be consciousness. This is a more life positive approach while the 'all is illusion' school is a more life negative approach. These can also be defined as the 'everything is empty' or 'everything is full' schools. Still another approach is that expounded in the Upanishads of 'not this, not this' (*neti neti*). This is yet another way to arrive at Purusha. It is simply declaring that everything that is not Purusha, pure consciousness, is not IT, so reject it. The reason why there are so many different approaches to Purusha is that Purusha is unknowable.

"That Purusha who is ever-present, consciousness and pure goes on creating charming objects for the senses

even when they are asleep. Purusha is Brahman, Purusha is called the immortal. All worlds are fixed on Him, none can transcend Him, He is That."
Katha Upanishad 2.2.8

Prakriti – Latent Matter

Purusha cannot manifest anything because it has no qualities that are related to matter. Being unknown it is devoid of the potential to manifest. Therefore, it needs a partner to manifest itself. Without a partner Purusha remains latent as pure beingness, or pure consciousness. In Samkhya the next principle of creation is called *Prakriti*, latent matter, or potential matter. Samkhya states that Purusha, for no reason, begins to reflect on itself. From this process of reflection Prakriti (latent matter) is born and begins to interact with Purusha (consciousness). All of this happens simultaneously, the reflection of pure consciousness on itself, resulting in latent matter, who then begins to interact with its source, pure consciousness. Hence, the 'play' or interaction of pure consciousness and matter is the fundamental cause of the manifestation. It has no reason to begin, nor does it have any goal. The Upanishads say that there is no goal of the creation; if there is a reason it could be for Purusha to experience itself. Being alone (mono) Purusha cannot know itself, as that requires two (dual) to exist. Hence, with the arrival of Prakriti dualism comes into being.

Prakriti is the actual source of the material manifestation. Prakriti is feminine in nature and is often referred to as Nature itself. In our language we could call Prakriti the power of Mother Nature. In Sanskrit another name of Prakriti is *Shakti* – the pure, latent, creative energy of creation. Prakriti, like Purusha, has three main attributes or qualities that form the basis of all creation. In Sanskrit they are called the three *Gunas*. Guna can be translated as attribute, or quality, literally it means to bind or hold together. Hence, everything that is in the creation has a mix of these three attributes.

The Gunas are often misunderstood and classified as being 'good or bad'. This is missing completely their role in creation. Tamas, the quality of darkness and decay is what allows new growth and creation. It allows life to end, the night to come and for us to fall asleep at night. Actually the physical universe depends on the Tamas principle of Prakriti as it represents the more solid, dense aspect of creation and eventually the five elements.

At this time it is important to interject a new concept that is important throughout the study of Samkhya or any of the ancient disciplines. The universe is multidimensional. Trying to give a fixed meaning to any of the principles will result in a misunderstanding because the meanings change according to the dimension being spoken of or experienced. This is a key point of effectively using Samkhya as a tool of understanding Ayurveda. This is also the most commonly misunderstood point I find when teaching others. Hence, looking at any of the attributes, or Gunas, changes enormously depending on the dimension.

For example, let's use the illustration of Tamas, the attribute of darkness, obscurity, and inertia. On the cosmic level matter derives itself from Tamas, on the level of the cosmic mind Tamas manifests as obscurity of Purusha, a veiling effect of the source of the cosmic mind. On the level of the individual mind Tamas presents itself as the idea of separation through veiling the cosmic mind (Mahat). Tamas becomes responsible for form as the manifestation begins to take shape in matter. The inertia allows the matter to solidify out of gaseous, heated forms. In the human body it allows for sleep and rest. In the human mind it caused delusion, depression, perversion, violence and addiction.

Therefore, looking at any attribute (Guna) of the manifestation without first defining what dimension is being addressed will lead to misunderstanding and a wrong interpretation. This is perhaps the most important point in understanding the Samkhya explanation of creation when learning Ayurveda.

Their names are Sattva, Rajas, and Tamas, or purity, action and inertia. They are described as follows:

GUNA	Cosmic Qualities	Mental Qualities	In Creation
Sattva	Purity, light, clarity, flexibility, harmony, virtue, luminous	Creativity, flexibility compassion, kindness, open, loving, caring, intelligent, humanitarian	Development
Rajas	Active, movement, dynamic, force, abrupt, distraction, impulse, turbulence, dispersing	Direct, aggressive, motivated, goal seeking, angry, controlling	Dispersing
Tamas	Inertia, darkness, obscurity, rigid, fixed, dull, heavy, solid, obstructing, matter	Delusion, dullness, stupidity, manipulating, violent, deceiving, dishonest, depression	Degeneration

As we have seen so far Prakriti, latent matter, exists as a potential. In and of itself it is not materialized, it is the potential of matter. That potential exists in three primary attributes, also latent. Prakriti comes into being through the subtle movement of Purusha, pure consciousness. Purusha is the conscious intelligent principle of the universe which, when combined with latent matter, begins the process of manifestation through the three attributes (Triguna) of Prakriti. The three qualities of Purusha, Satcitanand, are present in all aspects of the creation and in all three of the attributes of Prakriti.

"One should know that Prakriti is surely Māyā and that the great Purusha is the ruler of Māyā. This whole universe is truly pervaded by the appearance of creation."
Shetāshvatara Upanishad, 4.10

Mahat – The Cosmic Mind

The union of pure consciousness with pure creative energy gives birth to universal mind or *Mahat*. This next level or dimension of the creation manifests the cosmic principle of intelligence. Every future dimension or level of creation must have the principle of intelligence because Mahat symbolizes this quality of nature. While the Purusha represents pure, un-manifested consciousness, Mahat represents that consciousness manifested as intelligence. Through the process of manifestation this cosmic intelligence is no longer observed as 'pure'. This is one of the primary differences between Mahat and Purusha. Yet Mahat, as the first cosmic principle, is present in all creation and is omnipotent, or all pervading.

Prakriti, Nature as pure energy, gives its quality of existing to Mahat. Without Prakriti the cosmic mind would not be able to manifest because it is Prakriti that gives form to all things. Additionally, the three attributes of Prakriti begin to take form in Mahat. Therefore, if Mahat contains the three attributes of Prakriti it must also contain the three qualities of Purusha. Mahat is actually born from the three Gunas (attributes) of Prakriti, specifically rajas, the attribute of action and creation though movement. At this stage of the development of creation there is no concept of the individual. Up until this state there is only the sense of oneness, of unity.

Ahamkara – The Sense of 'I'

After the dimension of cosmic mind the creation begins to divide itself into separate manifestations. The beginning of this process is the *Ahamkara* or sense of 'I'. This refers to the development of the individualized concept. Everything following the Ahamkara in creation has a sense of being separate from its source. On one hand this sense causes great anguish and suffering. On the other hand it causes the diversification that makes the world rich in both name and form.

The anguish and suffering come from the sense of being separated from the cosmic mind, the joy of being in communion with Satcitanand, or Being, Consciousness, Bliss – the manifestation of Purusha through Prakriti and Mahat. All human suffering can be traced to this diversification, to this change in dimensions. Yet, this same diversification allows for the infinite variety in nature and its manifestation. By this process of separation from the cosmic mind the creation become infinitely rich and full.

The Ahamkara is that dimension when the individual comes into being. It is often translated as 'ego'. This description is deceptive and not entirely correct. Ahamkara has little to do with the Freudian concept of ego because it is far larger in conception. However, it is correct to say that the concept of Ahamkara includes the notion of the Freudian ego. The Ahamkara represents all diversification in the creation where the ego of Freud is concerned only with the individual conceptualization of the human being. Ahamkara is concerned with the whole universe and the basic principle of separateness.

The Ahamkara is also not the same as the Freudian ego even where the individual human is concerned. The Sanskrit word Ahamkara can be translated as 'that which fabricates the 'I'. The Upanishads often call the Ahamkara 'the I thought'. Both of these definitions refer to a development before the ego. They refer to the basic sense of beingness that is the foundation of the mind and all its mental and psychological functions. According to Samkhya the Ahamkara or 'I' is the foundation of the whole psychology. The sense of 'I' or separation needs to be there before the ego can exist.

Buddhi – The Individual Intellect

The *Buddhi* arrives in the manifestation with the diversification of Ahamkara. It is not part of the cosmic Samkhya system, rather is part of human development. The moment an individual human exists the potential of Buddhi is manifest. Buddhi, or intellect, does not exist in other forms of life. It is the Buddhi, or reasoning mind, which separates the human being from the animal kingdom. However, according to the Samkhya the intellect only exists as a potential – each individual has to developing it themselves. Otherwise the intellect remains dormant.

This then gives enormous freedom to the process of creation – the freedom to remain as a two-legged animal or to become a human being. This is determined by the use of the Buddhi – the reasoning mind. If the primary factor separating humans from animals is a faculty that is left unused then how can that being be called truly human? The Samkhya is not a fatalistic system – nature provides for full freedom on all levels of the creation, this is most apparent in the level of human potential.

The Buddhi actually comes directly from the Mahat – the cosmic mind. It is our own little piece of the cosmic or divine mind. It is the highest quality given to the human beings. However, it cannot manifest without the presence of Ahamkara, the sense of being an individual. Only through the diversification of the universal into the individual can a dimension be opened for Buddhi to exist. The name 'Buddhi' comes from the same Sanskrit root as 'Buddha' – from bud meaning 'to know'.

Levels of Buddhi

Level	Guna (Attribute)	Relation to Intellect
Higher	Sattva	Discriminating, humanitarian, feeling
Middle	Rajas	Logical, critical, reasoning, scientific
Lower	Tamas	Dogmatic, fixed, rigid concepts

The Buddhi is usually translated as 'intellect' or intellectual function. Attention should be brought to the fact that 'Buddhi' is much greater in scope that these concepts allow. The Buddhi can perhaps be better understood through looking at the three levels it functions on. On its highest level it is the power of conscious discrimination, which is feeling, caring and sensitive. This is the domain of Sattva (purity) in the Buddhi. The second level of Buddhi is the Rajasic (active) level. This relates to the logical, reasoning, dry critical aspect of Buddhi. This is the domain of modern science and is the part of Buddhi that is worshipped by modern society. However, it is insensitive to nature and life due to its dominance of Rajasic, dispersing energy. The lowest level of the Buddhi relates to the dogmatic, fixed intellect that holds on rigid fixed intellectual concepts. The following chart gives an overview of Buddhi.

Manas – The Individual Mind

After the concept of the individual, Ahamkara, the universe is in multiplicity. This gives rise to the 'Mind', or *Manas*. In this sense the word 'Mind' refers to several levels of function. Manas, or Mind, is not just thinking and is certainly not reasoning which is the middle domain of Buddhi. Manas is comparable to our whole psychology. It is more of a field, a thing, than an abstraction. The Mind, or Manas, has form and can be observed – thus it can be treated as an object. The treatment of the mind as an object in the Ayurvedic tradition provides the possibility to transform the psychology as it is an observable object. This is the subject of later lessons.

Manas is the feeling, thinking, emotional mind and also that part of the mind which is conditioned by family, friends, city, country and race. Manas is the part of the mind that modern psychology is primarily concerned with. It is the part we are the most aware of in our own minds. It is also the most unstable as it is influenced directly by the senses and outer environment. It is the part of the psychology, which receives outside impressions and brings them into the mind – this is why it can be conditioned. It is also common to the animal kingdom.

Manas is our daily thinking mind. It allows us to function on a 'normal' level and relates to both our environment and other people. If the Manas is disturbed or traumatized in some manner then the other aspects of the mind suffer in both function and interrelationship. Manas is our individual door to reality because it is an organ of both reception and expression.

"The mind (Manas) is superior to the senses; the intellect (Buddhi) is superior to the mind; Mahat is superior to the intellect; Prakriti is superior to Mahat. Superior to Prakriti is the Purusha who is all pervasive and is without worldly attributes, knowing Purusha a man becomes free and attains immortality."
Katha Upanishad, 2.3.7-8

Tanmatras – Matter in Subtle Form

Until this moment the universe has remained in a subtle, divers state. The principle of differentiation has come into being (Ahamkara) along with the ability to perceive it (Manas). Now, the next dimension of the universe arrives as a five-fold division of subtle matter. The universe is still without solid form at this point. One can say that 'name' or classification has arisen with the mind, but not yet 'form' in a subtle or solid sense. With this five-fold division of matter subtle form comes into existence.

In Sanskrit the word *Tanmatra* can be translated as 'primal measure' or 'root action'. It is the cause of all solid matter as we know it. The Tanmatras are potentials of matter – they themselves are not matter – they are the potential of matter. They are directly responsible for the five main divisions of matter, or categories of matter. At this point in the creation the Prana divides itself five-fold as well. It can be argued that the Tanmatras are primarily the division of Prana as it becomes more dense or solid. Hence, the Tanmatras are a dynamic force that are driven by the five divisions of Prana.

The Tanmatras represent the five states of matter in a pure form. The scriptures describe these states of matter as – a field or space, movement of gases, transformation, liquid or cohesion and lastly, solid. All of the manifested universe can be put into one of these five categories. The Tanmatras represent these five states of matter in their purest form. In order for matter to come into being there needs to be an interaction between these different states – the dimension of the Tanmatras is before this interaction.

The Five States of Matter (Panchamahabhuta)

On this dimension form comes into being. Prior to this level nothing has existed in a concrete, stable, solid manner. The five primary states of matter or *Pancha Maha Bhutani* come into being because of the previous dimension – they cannot exist without it. These states interact causing all matter to manifest from this interaction. These states of matter represents categories – all matter can fit into one of these five categories. Unfortunately, they are usually translated as the 'Five Elements', which gives a very erroneous idea of what they represent. The word 'element' has little to do with the alive, interactive state of matter that is meant by the Sanskrit word Bhutani. There is a lesson on this subject because Ayurveda is based on the concept of Pancha Maha Bhuta.

The Five Forms of Reception (Jnanendriyani)

Once matter comes into existence there needs to be some means to perceive it. The ancients observed that the five forms of matter were received respectively by five sense organs (*Jnanendriyani*). These five forms of reception receive the name and form (classification and structure) of the five principle categories of manifestation.

They are often called the five 'sense organs' in the ancient texts of Samkhya and the Upanishads. Yet, the Sanskrit word is far more potent in depth and meaning. Jnanendriyani, means something closer to 'the potential to receive, on all levels, experiences of the physical, mental and subtle world'. These five forms of reception are mainly concerned with how the psychology receives impressions and information into Manas (the mind) from the outside manifestation or material world.

The Five Forms of Expression (Karmendriyas)

Just as there is a need for the reception of the manifestation so too there is a need for the interaction with this universe through expression. Hence, there is a counterpart of expression that correspond to the five forms of reception; these are the five forms of action or the *Karmendriyas*. Ultimately, the Upanishads state that Pure Consciousness, Purusha, manifests in order to interact with itself. This is sometimes called the divine play or 'Lila'. Therefore, the means of both reception and expression are necessary for the Purusha to experience itself.

Without some means to express the circle of creation is not complete. There has to be a way to express both the joy or pain of the impressions received in the manifestation. This allows the freedom to respond according to the attribute, or Guna, that is predominating in the mental dimension. If the attributes are of a pure nature (Sattva) then the expressions will be creative, beautiful and harmonious to the situation. If the attributes dominate in the psychology are extroverted (Rajas) then the expressions will be dynamic, aggressive, and goal orientated. If the attribute that is dominating the mind is languid (Tamas) then the force of inertia prevails through expression of negative emotions, violence and even the lack of expression itself.

Tables of Relationships

State of Matter	Reception	Expression
Space – Ether	Sound – Ears	Speech – Mouth
Movement – Wind	Touch – Skin	Grip or Hold – Hands
Heat – Fire	Sight – Eyes	Motion – Feet
Liquid – Water	Taste – Tongue	Emission – Urino-Genital
Solid – Earth	Smell – Nose	Elimination – Anus

For more information on the subject of Samkhya Darshana you can read my book called *The Psychology of Transformation in Yoga* which goes into detail on the application of Samkhya in Yoga, Ayurveda and Jyotish.

The Samkhya View of Creation

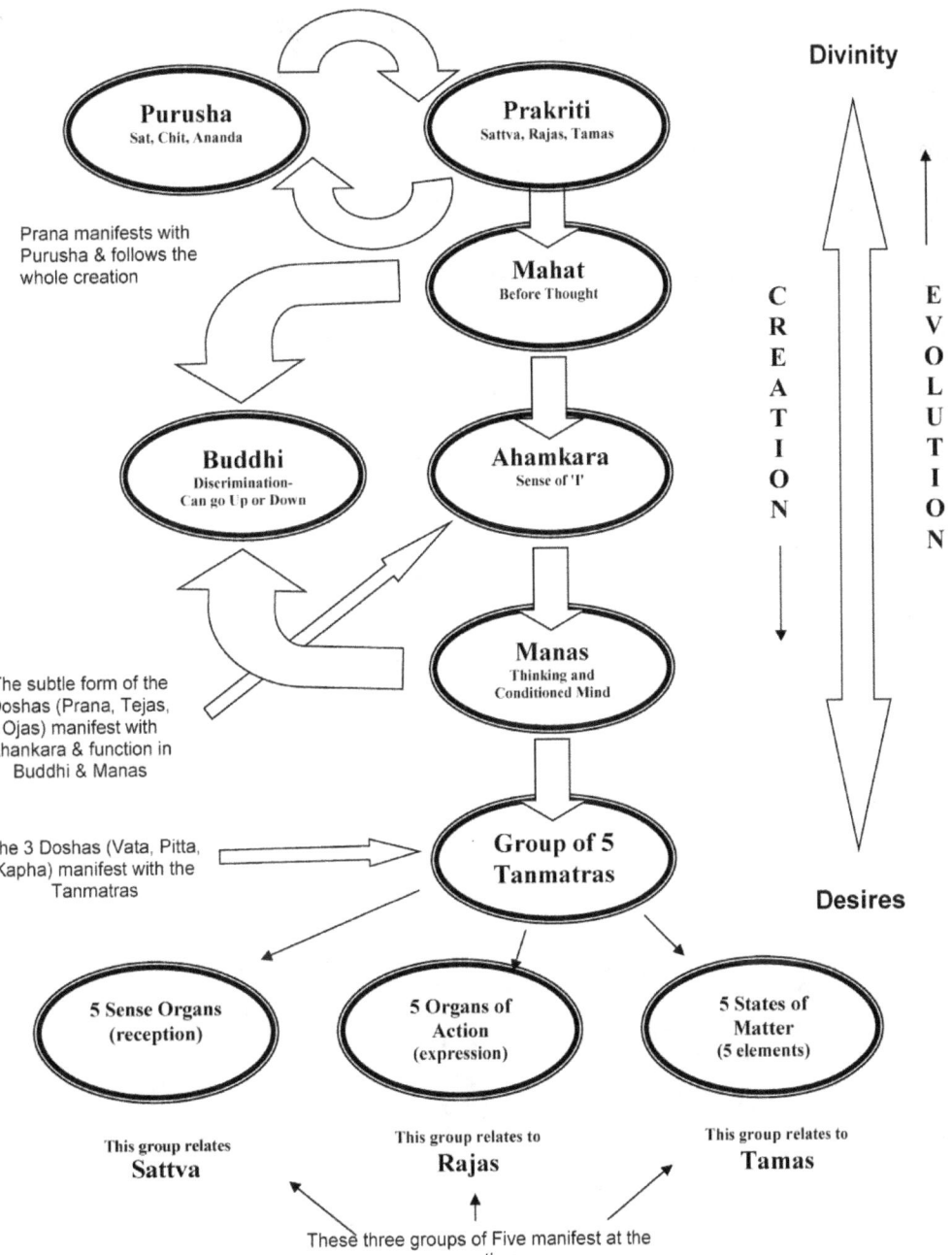

Chapter One Study Questions

1. Why are there six Darshanas in Indian thinking?

2. Which three are the most important for the study of Ayurveda?

3. What is the most important idea in the Samkhya Darshana?

4. Why is Samkhya called a philosophy?

5. Why is it important to learn the Samkhya vision of creation?

6. What is a Tattva?

7. Where does Purusha come from?

8. What is Ahamkara?

9. What are the Tanmatras?

10. What is the reason there are 5 sense organs and 5 motor organs?

CHAPTER TWO
HISTORY OF AYURVEDA

The origins of Indian history are obscured by time. Oral tradition in India tells us that the basis of Indian culture is presented in the Vedas. These are four groups of verses or hymns are named as Rig Veda, Yajur Veda, Sama Veda and Atharva Veda. They are known as 'Apaurusheya', meaning that they have not evolved from a human mind, rather they are conceived by the divine mind or Atman. They are eternal and have no beginning or end. Together they form what is called the 'Sanatana Dharma', or the 'eternal truth'. Thus, the Veda cannot be limited historically to any period of history or pre-history as understood by historians who formed the history of India in the colonial era.

My teacher told me that the current Vedic era is more than 40,000 years old. It is important to understand that India is an oral tradition culture - not a written tradition culture. The history of Ayurveda is shrouded in mystery because Indian culture felt that writing was an inferior method of record keeping. Indian's are well known to be able to memorize 40,000 to 200,000 *sutras* (verses or hymns) and recite then flawlessly with perfect Sanskrit intonation and meter. A master of this art can not only recite the verses perfectly, but can also recite them backwards from the end of the text to the beginning flawlessly!

Because of this particular view of learning and recording history very little has been written about ancient Indian by the Indian's themselves. Unfortunately, some deluded Western scholars try to date Indian and Ayurvedic texts by the style of written Sanskrit. This is a major flaw when trying to understand the historical origins of anything in India. Writing is a relatively new development in India and hence it limits the Veda, Ayurveda and other knowledge to the last few thousand years. The real problem is that the Christian Ego that forms Western culture cannot admit to a culture that was civilized 20,000 or 30,000 years before the first European culture. To even give a moment of validity to Indian oral tradition would mean that the Bible and Christian chronology is incorrect. The Western Ego cannot abide this so finds any method to discount the alive oral tradition of India.

We do know a great deal about ancient India from the Chinese and Persians who were great writers and historians. Thus, most of what we have in recorded information about ancient India and Ayurveda come from either merchants or scholars, not necessarily doctors. Judging from the records of the Chinese we can surmise that Ayurveda began to be formulated into public health care prior to 3,000 BC. This is supported by archeological discoveries in the last decade that have found cities more than 7,000 years old that have indoor plumbing, attached bathrooms and sewer systems to evacuate waste.

In the history of medicine it is clear that the most important discovery for the health of humanity has not been vaccines, but rather sanitation. Therefore, it is illogical to assume that public health of large, ancient cites was an arbitrary manifestation of luck. Moreover, it is clearly stated in the oldest Ayurvedic text, the Caraka Samhita, that Ayurveda came into being from the concern of the wise men of the period who saw the grouping of people into city environments as a major concern for general health and welfare. Ayurveda developed from the physical and sociological needs of humanity in that time and place.

The word *Ayurveda* comes from two words: Ayur which comes the from the root *ayus* - meaning 'to live' or 'life'; and from Veda which comes from the root *vid* - 'to know' or 'knowledge'. Together these form the word Ayurveda or the knowledge of life. Literally, ayur in this context means longevity, so the best definition we can use for Ayurveda would be: the 'knowledge of longevity' or the 'knowledge of life'.

Divine Origins

Ayurveda has divine origins according to oral tradition. It is stated that Ayurveda has no beginning or end. Divine Knowledge has no beginning or ending. Ayurveda resides in the eternal cosmic intelligence, or Atman. Ayurveda has been imparted to the saints and sages (Rishis) who gained the knowledge through meditation and interaction with the gods.

The oral tradition of Ayurveda tells us that it originated in the Atman as a thought in the mind of Brahma, the creator. He conveyed it to Daksha Prajapati. From Prajapati the entire knowledge was passed on to the Ashwini Kumaras who were the twin god physicians of the Devas or divine beings in the Devaloka (commonly translated as gods and paradise - however, not as in the Christian sense of the words).

The twin gods Ashwini Kumaras offered Ayurveda to Lord Indra, the king of gods in Vedic mythology. Indra then taught three great physicians as his disciples; Rishi Bharadvaja, Rishi Kashyapa and Rishi Dhanvantari. Indra presented Ayurveda as the *tri-sutras* to Rishi Bharadvaja, which are—*etiology* or the science of the causes of disease, *symptomatology* or the study and interpretation of symptoms, and clinical treatments.

Vedic hymns associated with Ayurveda appear in the Rig Veda. These verses of Rig Veda, the earliest source of Ayurveda, refer to panchamahabhuta (five basic categories of matter) and the three doshas or primary forces of Prana / Vata (air), Agni / (fire) and soma / Kapha (water) as comprising the basic principles of Ayurveda.

However, it is in the Atharva Veda, the youngest of the four Vedas, that one finds many references to medicine. The Atharva Veda is not only an important source of knowledge about practical life, religion and magic, but also includes descriptions of anatomy, medical treatments and explanations of certain diseases. Sometime prior to 10,000 BC the Sama Veda and Yajur Veda - the second and third Vedas - came into being. Chanting of mantras and performance of rituals were, respectively, dealt in these two Vedas. After 10,000 BC the Atharva Veda was authored. Ayurveda is an *upaveda* (subsection) of this Veda. Thus, it is considered a sub-branch of Vedic knowledge and is therefore sacred. This Vedic period of Ayurveda originated from the three Rishis that where taught by Indra.

Rishi Bharadwaj had one primary disciple named Atreya Punarvasu. This disciple Atreya Punarvasu is the origin of the most ancient Ayurvedic text, the Caraka Samhita. Atreya's main disciple was called Acharya Agnivesha. He formulated the main Ayurvedic text of internal medicine, which was revised and compiled by his student, Acharya Caraka. Therefore, the text is known today as the Caraka Samhita.

Dhanvantari is the god of medicine in India and is considered to be an incarnation of Vishnu - the preserver of humanity. Rishi Sushruta, was the renowned disciple of Dhanvantari and he wrote the second most important text on Ayurveda, known as the Sushruta Samhita. It is the most important text on surgery and comprises the knowledge about prosthetic surgery to replace limbs, cosmetic surgery, and even brain surgery. He is famed for his innovation of cosmetic surgery on the nose or rhinoplasty; a method still taught and used today.

One branch of the six Indian Darshana (lit., 'a way to see reality') called *Samkhya Darshana* states that there are 24 elements (*Tattva*), all of which constitute the foundation of gross matter: earth, water, fire, air and ether. These five states of matter (*panchamahabhuta*) in different combinations constitute the three doshas - Vata dosha (air and ether), Pitta dosha (fire and water) and Kapha dosha (earth and water). The panchamahabhuta and the *Tridosha* theories are the guiding factors of Ayurveda as a therapeutic science. The concepts codified in the Samkhya Darshana are found in the Vedas and are an integrated part of Ayurveda.

Though Ayurveda came into being as an independent upaveda of the Atharva Veda, it has close links with other Vedas also. The Yajur Veda, which recommends rituals to pacify the panchamahabhutas in a view to heal both the Cosmic Being (*Atman*) and the individual soul (*Jiva Atman*), is related to Ayurveda in its principles and regulations of lifestyle. The upaveda called Dhanur Veda (martial arts) and Ayurveda both refer to each other in the treatment of *marmas* or sensitive points in the body.

Recorded History

Around 2,000 BC to 3,000 BC Ayurveda was delineated into to two distinct schools: the Atreya school - The School of Internal Medicine; and the Dhanvantari school -The School of Surgery. This made Ayurveda a more systematically classified medical science. These two schools codified their teachings into two texts; the Caraka Samhita and Sushruta Samhita. In this process of codification they were taken from the oral tradition and written out sometime between 2,000 BC and 1,000 BC.

Though it had been practiced all along, it was around this time that Ayurveda was developed as an independent Veda. Eight branches or divisions of Ayurveda where clarified and called *Ashtanga Ayurveda*:

1. Kayachikitsa (Internal Medicine)
2. Shalakya Tantra (Treatment of Head, Ophthalmology & Otolaryngology)
3. Shalya Tantra (Surgery)
4. Agada Tantra (Toxicology)
5. Bhuta Vidya (Psychiatry)

6. Kaumarabhritya (Pediatrics)
7. Rasayana (Rejuvenation or anti-aging)
8. Vajikarana (Science of fertility).

Around 500 AD, Acharya Vagbhatta compiled the third major treatise on Ayurveda, Ashtanga Hridaya. It contains knowledge comprising the two previous schools of Ayurveda—the school of internal medicine (Caraka) and the school of surgery (Sushruta). In and of itself it is not entirely a new presentation of Ayurveda. The author, Acharya Vagbhatta, made an analysis of both Caraka and Sushruta and presented them in a logical manner that is more accessible than the earlier texts.

These three ancient scriptures (*Samhita*) - Caraka Samhita, Sushruta Samhita and Ashtanga Hridaya are known as *Brihattrayi* (Major Triad) and they form the most important knowledge of Ayurvedic medicine at present.

In later centuries important information about pathology, diagnosis, medicinal herbs, minerals and food was recorded in three texts named: Madhava Nidana, Bhava Prakasha and Ashtanga Sharangdha. Together they are known as *Laghutrayi* (Minor Triad) and form the second main group of text books on Ayurvedic medicine.

From 500 AD to 1900 AD, sixteen major Nighantus or supplementary texts on Ayurveda like Dhanvantari Nighantu, Raja and Shaligram among others were written incorporating new drugs, expansion in applications, discarding of old drugs and identification of substitutes.

Historical evidence shows that Ayurveda had influenced almost all the medical systems of the ancient world. The Egyptians learnt about Ayurveda long before the invasion of Alexander in the 4th century BC through their sea-trade with India. Greeks and Romans come to know about it after the invasion of Alexander the Great. The Unani form of medical tradition came out of this interaction between Persian, Greek and Indian cultures. From 100 AD to 300 AD Ayurveda spread to the East through Buddhism and greatly influenced the Tibetan and Chinese systems of medicine. Around 323 BC, Nagarjuna, the great monastic of Mahayana Buddhism and an authority on Ayurveda wrote a commentary on the Sushruta Samhita. In 800 AD Ayurveda was translated into Arabic. The two Islamic physicians Avicenna and Razi Serapion, who helped form the European tradition of medicine, strictly followed Ayurveda. Even, Paracelsus, considered to be the father of the modern Western medicine followed the precepts of Ayurveda.

From around 1000 AD on Ayurveda suffered first from multiple Mogul invasions followed by the British Empire which actively suppressed Ayurvedic practice. During centuries of colonial rule, Ayurvedic institutions were not officially supported. In fact, most Ayurvedic practices were actively suppressed. Much important clinical and theoretical knowledge was lost during this time period. Experts in the various approaches of Ayurveda—specialists in herbal medicines, purifications procedures, diagnosis and many other modalities—lost contact with each other. Most significantly, the central role of consciousness, of meditation and other mental techniques, was temporarily eclipsed due to the Western European influence. At one point during British occupation Ayurvedic doctors had their hands cut off if they were found to be practicing Ayurveda.

In the 10th and 12th centuries when India was occupied by Muslim invaders they brought their own medicine, Unani, a blend of Islamic medicine and Greek medicine. Ayurveda's popularity declined in this period. Unani and Ayurveda, which have mutually influenced each other from 400 BC to 1200 AD are both practiced today in India. In the 13th or 14th century Sarngadhara Samhita was written by Acharya Vagbhatta, which introduced new treatments and described new syndromes. During the period of King Akbar, the liberal Muslim ruler, Ayurveda flourished with a free exchange of ideas between Western and Indian physicians. During the British occupation, Ayurveda declined and western medicine was promoted. This was carried out through brutal repression by British agents who cut off the hands of practicing *Vaidyas* (doctors) in order to stop the use of Ayurveda. In the late 20th century once again the interest of Ayurveda increased. In 1947, when India gained independence from the British, Ayurveda was recognized as an official form of medicine along with allopathy, homeopathy, naturopathy, unani, siddha and yoga therapy.

When India became politically independent in 1947, Ayurveda was in disarray, with widely varying standards of quality and conflicts of opinion. A new spirit of national pride stimulated its revival. In 1971, Ayurveda was made part of India's official state healthcare system, which had until then been exclusively Western. Still, Ayurvedic experts felt that Ayurveda was not what it once had been. Some areas of Ayurveda that were recorded in ancient texts are essentially unavailable or missing.

The current situation for Ayurveda in India is hopeful. For centuries Ayurveda has been cut from its holistic Spiritual, Mind, Body roots by Western powers. The current interest in Ayurveda by Europeans and Americans (North and South) has sparked a revival movement. Unfortunately, the major problem facing Ayurveda in India is the outdated educational system. The curriculum established in 1947 to 1949 has never been updated and mixes almost half of allopathic studies in with Ayurveda. The result is a mix of neither Ayurveda nor allopathy. The Health Department needs to review and update the status of Ayurveda so that it can live up to its potential in India.

The Sutrasthana section of the Caraka Samhita, says;
"*The three - body, mind and soul - are like a tripod, the world is sustained by their combination; they constitute the substratum of everything. The combination of these three is Purusha. This is the subject matter of Ayurveda for which these teachings have been revealed.*" (CS.SU.1.46-47)

The three classical texts of Ayurveda

Caraka Samhita

The Caraka Samhita is considered to be the most ancient and authoritative writing on Ayurveda available today. This Samhita contains 8,400 metrical verses in Sanskrit. It also explains the logic and philosophy on which this system of medicine is based. The detailed biography of the sage Caraka is not known. Interestingly, it is not an original writing of a single person. Like all Vedic knowledge it is a continuation and renewal of that eternal body of knowledge. In fact, Caraka had rewrote the Agnivesa Samhita (an edited version of the Atreya Samhita). The currently available form of the Caraka Samhita was again rewritten by sage Drdhabala (about 400 AD) long after sage Caraka was dead.

Caraka followed the Atreya School of Internal Medicine, which predominantly deals with treatments through internal and external application of medicine. Though the Samhita contains all the theoretical knowledge of Ayurveda it`s focus is on healing the body, mind and soul of a patient in the minimum invasive manner that is called *Kayachikitsa*. Hence, he placed great emphasis on the diagnostic part of the treatment. He identified eight stages of a disease from its inception to the culmination. Caraka also laid great emphasis on the timing and manner of the collection of medicinal plants.

According to Caraka, science is dependent upon yukti - a quality of the intellect that enables it to perceive phenomena brought into existence by a multiplicity of causes. Thus, it`s not surprising that much of the treatise of Caraka Samhita is in the form of a symposium wherein groups of Ayurveda scholars take up a series of topics for discussion. This indicates that the science of Ayurveda is a product of constant verification, fine-tuning and authentication by an active community of physicians. The Samhita explains the gradual development of the fetus within the womb in minutes that equals the modern medical version in accuracy and insights.

Caraka sought to correct the element of fire or Agni in the digestive function. He sought to alter the chemical processes in the cells by purification methods and medicinal application. From a greater perspective Caraka laid emphasis for health and longevity to strike a balance between one`s physical and spiritual being.

Sushruta Samhita

Sushruta renowned as the father of plastic surgery, wrote the most authentic text on the practice of Ayurvedic surgery. He represents the Dhanvantari School of Surgery. His Samhita discusses in detail how to perform prosthetic surgery to replace limbs, cosmetic surgery on nose and on other parts of the body, cesarean operations, and setting of compound fractures. Sushruta`s original work seems to have been revised and supplemented by Nagarjuna between the third and fourth centuries AD. The style Sushruta Samhita is both prose and poetry with poetry being the greater portion. This work, also, is said to be a redaction of oral material passed down verbally from generation to generation.

This branch of medicine is believed to have arisen in part from the exigencies of dealing with the effects of war. The epic Ramayana, mentions remarkable feats of surgery having taken place in the past.

This work is unique in that it discusses blood in terms of the fourth doshic principle. This work is the first to enumerate and discuss the Pitta subtypes. Sushruta details about 125 surgical instruments used by him mostly made of stone, wood and other such natural materials. The Sushruta Samhita presents many innovations in Ayurvedic surgery. Use of shalaka—meaning foreign body (here, rods or a probe etc.) is mentioned by Sushruta. Some of the classifications in anatomy found in the Sushruta Samhita have not been discovered by the modern medical science.

Sushruta has discussed about 72 diseases of the eye. He has stipulated drug therapy for various types of conjunctivitis and glaucoma along with surgical procedures of the removal of cataract, pterygium, diseases of ear, nose and throat. In fact he is the first surgeon in medical history who systematically and elaborately dealt with anatomical structure of eye.

Ashtanga Hridaya

Ashtanga Hridaya is accepted as the third major treatise on Ayurveda. It was written around 500 AD. Rishi Vagbhatta compiled this Samhita. It contained knowledge comprising the two schools of Ayurveda—the school of surgery and the school of internal medicine.

There is another similar work called the Ashtanga Samgraha belonging to the same period. It is slightly bigger in size than the Ashtanga Hridaya, and is written in verse form whereas the later text was in prose form. It is believed either there are two works by a person or two persons with the same name. However, both the works came into being after the Caraka and Sushruta Samhitas.

The Ashtanga Hridaya primarily deals with Kayachikitsa besides, discussing in detail about various surgical treatments. The Kapha subtypes are first listed and described in this Samhita, completing exhaustive explanation of Vata, Pitta, Kapha with their five subtypes.

Ashtanga Hridaya seems to emphasize on the physiological aspect of the body rather than the spiritual aspects of it unlike its counterparts: the Caraka and Sushruta Samhitas. Despite that, the quality and range of its discussions about Ayurveda makes it a work worthy to study. Current tradition in India states that a student should begin with study of the Ashtanga Hridaya and terminate with the study of the Caraka or Sushruta Samhitas.

Chapter Two Study Questions

1. Why is it hard to pinpoint dates historically in Ayurveda?

2. What cultures keep records of the most ancient periods of Ayurvedic development?

3. What has been the most important discovery for the health of humanity?

4. Ayurveda is said to have divine origins; which person did Brahma teach first?

5. What does upaveda mean?

6. What does Ashtanga Ayurveda mean?

7. Who started the school of surgery in Ayurveda?

8. What are the *Laghutrayi* (Minor Triad)?

9. Which invading culture cut off the hands of practicing Vaidyas in India?

10. Which Samhita is the best to learn from first?

CHAPTER THREE
THE TWENTY ATTRIBUTES AND FIVE ELEMENTS

In order to recognize matter there is a logical system of identification in India. This system is related to the dualistic nature of manifestation and represents the 'masculine/feminine' or 'negative/positive' aspects of polarity in creation. The system uses the qualities or "attributes" (Guna) of any substance to understand it. These "attributes" exist in ten pairs and all objects or states can be placed in one of these pairs. It is not an extensive list as other pairs can be found, but these are regarded as the most primary and important when understanding the qualities of creation.

These twenty qualities (called the *Gurvadi Guna*) are subdivisions of the three Gunas (attributes) of Prakriti, or the Maha Guna: Sattva, Rajas and Tamas. From the interrelationship of these three primal attributes arise the ten pairs of opposites. Hence they are directly related to Prakriti, latent matter. They are used specifically to classify matter on all levels. In Ayurveda they are used to understand both the structural and functional aspects; e.g. the five states of matter and their controlling dosha.

The real key to practice Ayurvedic medicine is by using the Gurvadi Gunas in pathology, diagnosis and treatments. They need time to understand and memorize. Once this is done the clinical application of Ayurveda becomes much easier.

Below is a table that gives the ten pairs of attributes:

English	Sanskrit	English	Sanskrit
Cold	*Shita*	Hot	*Ushna*
Wet/ Oily	*Snigdha*	Dry	*Ruksha*
Heavy	*Guru*	Light	*Laghu*
Gross	*Sthula*	Subtle	*Sukshma*
Dense	*Sandra*	Flowing	*Drava/Shara*
Static	*Sthira*	Mobile	*Chala*
Dull/Low	*Manda*	Sharp/High	*Tikshna*
Soft	*Mridu*	Hard	*Kathina*
Smooth	*Slakahna*	Rough	*Khara*
Cloudy	*Picchila*	Clear	*Vishada*

According to classical texts this is how the twenty attributes relate to their source – the three Maha Guna (attributes) of Prakriti (matter).

Guna	Qualities
Sattva	Light, subtle, mobile, sharp, soft, smooth, clear
Rajas	Hot, gross, mobile, sharp, hard, rough, cloudy
Tamas	Cold, wet, heavy, gross, solid, static, dull, hard, rough, cloudy

All matter can be classified by using these ten pairs of opposites. They exist in all objects and situations of life. They can always be observed and used to understand the creation. They provide a working model of the subtle and observable universe. Through them we can understand the natural balance of nature that works through opposite forces to maintain equilibrium in the creation according to the Vedic perspective as seen by the *Rishis* or sages.

The principal way Ayurveda chooses therapies or therapeutic substances is through the "Twenty Attributes" or 20 Gunas. Using this model one can look at anything occurring in nature and describe its qualities. For example the weather today is rainy, cloudy, muggy and humid so I could describe today as – cool, wet, heavy, dense, static, somewhat dull, soft and cloudy or obscure. Or another example could be food, say an apple – cool, light, subtle, static and slightly rough.

This methodology is central to understanding Ayurvedic therapeutics. All of Ayurveda is based on observation. This is why it is so logical because one can readily see the results of correct or incorrect choices. Yet, it also provides a logical method for choosing anything from a climate that is suitable, to diet or herbal medicines. The only thing a practitioner has to do is observe the attributes dominant in the patient. For example, if a patient has dry skin you would choose substances that have the opposite quality – i.e., oil that is wet or increases humidity in the body. If the skin is dry and cold (Vata) the oil of choice would be warm or have a warming action.

Using this methodology does require the development of observation powers. In the past this was a universal sign of a good doctor, one who could look at you and understand what was happening to you. *This still is a universal sign of being a good doctor!* It is absolutely necessary that each practitioner develop this ability to recognize what attribute or qualities are dominating in the patient and their environment. A failure to do this will result in a completely mechanical approach to healing and your patient. Everything else is already written out for the practitioner. Ayurvedic books are full of the qualities of every substance commonly used today. The only effort a practitioner needs to make is to develop their own powers of observation and apply them!

The Twenty Attributes (Gurvadi Gunah)
- From the three Gunas come the twenty main attributes (ten pairs of opposites).
- They are positive and negative—the masculine and feminine of all forces in the universe.
- They are the *basis for the properties of all objects in nature* both material and mental.

Śita	Cold or cool	Uṣṇa	Hot
Guru	Heavy/Hard to digest	Laghu	Light/Easy to digest
Snigdha	Unctuous	Rūkṣa	Dry
Sthūla	Big/Thick/Gross	Sūkṣma	Minute/Thin/Subtle
Sthira	Steady/Static	Cala	Unsteady/Mobile
Sāñdra	Viscous/Dense	Drava/Sara	Flowing/Liquid/Spreading
Mañda	Slow/Dull/Moderate	Tīkṣṇa	Fast/Sharp/Penetrating
Mṛdu	Soft	Kaṭhiṇa	Hard
Ślakṣṇa	Smooth	Khara	Rough
Picchila	Gelatinous/Slimy/Opaque	Viśada	Non-slimy/Clear/Porous

Analysis of the Twenty Attributes

Śita ↓P ↑VK [Cold] Relates to ETHER, AIR, WATER, EARTH	**Uṣṇa ↑P ↓VK [Hot]** *Main attribute of PITTA* Relates to FIRE / PITTA
Snigdha ↑KP ↓V [Oily, Humid] *Main attribute of KAPHA* Relates to WATER / KAPHA	**Rūkṣa ↑V ↓K, mildly ↓P [Dry]** *Main attribute of VĀTA* Relates to AIR / VATA
Guru ↑K ↓V, mildly ↓P [Heavy] Relates to EARTH and WATER	**Laghu ↑V, mildly ↑P, ↓K [Light]** Relates to FIRE, AIR and ETHER
Sthūla ↑K ↓V, mildly ↓P [Gross] Relates to EARTH and WATER	**Sūkṣma ↑VP, ↓K [Subtle]** Relates to FIRE, AIR and ETHER
Sāñdra ↑K ↓VP [Viscous, Dense] Relates to EARTH	**Drava/Sara ↑PK, ↓V [Spreading]** Relates to FIRE and warm WATER
Sthira ↑K, ↓VP [Steady] Relates to EARTH and WATER	**Cala ↑VP, ↓K [Movement]** Relates to ETHER and AIR
Mañda ↑K, ↓VP [Dull, Slow, Low] Relates to EARTH and WATER	**Tīkṣṇa ↑VP, ↓K [Penetrating]** Relates to ETHER, AIR and FIRE
Mṛdu ↑KP, ↓V [Soft] Relates to WATER	**Kaṭhiṇa ↑V, ↓PK [Hard]** Relates to AIR and EARTH
Slakshna ↑KP, ↓V [Smooth] Relates to WATER	**Khara ↑V, ↓PK [Rough]** Relates to AIR and EARTH
Picchila ↑K, ↓VP [Mucilage] Relates to EARTH and WATER	**Viśada ↑VP, ↓K [Clear]** Relates to ETHER, AIR and FIRE

Attributes – Gunas – Elements – Doshas

	EARTH	WATER	FIRE	AIR	ETHER	V	P	K
COLD	X	X		XX	XXX	XX		X
WET/OILY		XXX					X	XX
HEAVY	XXX	XX					X	XX
GROSS	XXX	XX					X	XX
DENSE	XX	X					X	XX
STATIC	XX	X						XX
DULL	XX	X						XX
SOFT		XXX	XX				XX	X
SMOOTH		XX	X				X	XX
CLOUDY	XXX	XX	X				X	XX
HOT			XXX	XX	X		XX	
DRY	X		XX	XXX	X	XX		
LIGHT			X	XX	XXX	XX	X	
SUBTLE			X	XX	XXX	XX	X	
FLOWING		XX	XX			X	XX	
MOBILE				XXX	X	XX		
SHARP			X	XX	X	X	XX	
HARD	XXX			XX	X	XX		X
ROUGH	XXX			XX	X	X		
CLEAR				XX	XXX	X		

X = mild manifestation of attributes
XX = medium manifestation of attributes
XXX = strong manifestation of attributes

The Five States of Matter

The Samkhya system explains the manifestation of consciousness in a descending motion that results in physical matter. Prior to this physical level nothing has existed in a concrete, stable, solid manner. The five states of matter come into being because of the previous dimension – the *Tanmatra* – they cannot exist without it.

The ancient texts give the following analogy to the *Pancha Maha Bhutani* (five primary states of matter) to help the student comprehend their formation and function. "From the void of nothingness there arose a subtle movement of consciousness. As this movement became more concentrated various gaseous substances manifested. The movement of these gases caused friction, which began to transform the gases into humid condensation. This condensation began to solidify and create liquid as a cohesive substance. Finally, this liquid settled and solidified into solid matter."

The texts further state that 1/10 of space becomes gaseous, and 1/10 of gas becomes transformative heat, and 1/10 of heat becomes cohesive liquid, and 1/10 of liquid becomes solid. Therefore, solid matter contains a small part of each of the others which is why it is solid. It is the interaction of these states that allow for the manifestation to occur. Only space or ether remains pure and each of the other states has some portion of the previous states.

Ayurveda is based on the observation of nature and the interaction of consciousness that occurs in creation. The basis of these observations is that of matter itself which can be classified into five primary categories. The five primary categories of matter (*Pañcāmahābhūta*) form the basis of traditional Indian medicine. All of matter can be classified into one of the five following groups –

State of Matter	Attribute	Element (metaphoric)
Field	Space	Ether
Gaseous	Movement	Wind (Air)
Transformative	Heat	Fire
Liquid	Cohesive	Water
Density	Solid	Earth

In modern language the five primary states of matter are usually translated as the 'five elements'. This translation fails to convey the Sanskrit term, *Pañca māha bhūta*, which clearly means 'the five primary categories of substance'. Each category contains numerous sub-divisions of matter.

These states interact causing all matter to manifest from this interaction. These states of matter represents categories – all matter can fit into one of these five categories. Unfortunately, they are translated as the 'Five Elements', which gives a very erroneous idea of what they represent. The word 'element' has little to do with the alive, interactive state of matter that is meant by the Sanskrit word *Bhutani*.

These five states also manifest ideas and concepts – they are not limited to physical form, but also influence subtle form through the Tanmatras. This dimension is the dimension of alchemy and other ancient sciences like astrology. Possible relations of the subtle manifestation of conceptual thought as follows:

State of Matter	Conceptual Thought
Field	Connection, communication, unity
Gaseous	Movement, direction, penetration
Transformative	Transformation, light, perception
Liquid	Cohesion, binding, holding
Density	Solidity, stability

The five states of matter are the basis of all ancient sciences. They are the result of direct observation and can be experienced in life and observed directly. They are existential, experiential and experimental in nature. The whole universe is comprised of these states and comes into existence through their interaction. They are profound and require contemplation to comprehend, as they are also metaphoric for the various archetypes of nature as a whole.

Table of Relationships

State of Matter (5 elements)	Reception (5 sense organs)	Expression (5 motor organs)
Space – Ether	Sound – Ears	Speech – Mouth
Movement – Wind	Touch – Skin	Grip or Hold – Hands
Heat – Fire	Sight – Eyes	Motion – Feet
Liquid – Water	Taste – Tongue	Emission – Urino-Genital
Solid – Earth	Smell – Nose	Elimination – Anus

Locations of the Five Elements in the Body

Ether – Head, governing mind and senses, nervous system.
Wind – Heart, chest and arms, the center of the circulatory and respiratory systems.
Fire – Mid abdomen from its center the navel that relates to the digestive fire.
Water – Lower abdomen, hips, buttocks (where water and fat accumulate most, and site of urino-genital system).
Earth – Lower thighs to feet. Governs stability (e.g., to stand).

Actions of the Five Elements in the Body

Ether – Relates to space in the body and defines areas.
Wind – Relates to movement of all types, effort and breathing.
Fire – Relates to blood, urges like hunger and thirst (digestive system) and passion.
Water – Relates to plasma, urine, sweat, mucus and other liquid tissues.

Earth – Relates to bones, muscles, skin, hair, nails and other solid tissues.

Sequential Evolution of the Five Elements with an Analogy of Plant Growth

1. Akasha = uniform expansion

In a raw form the seed is very hard, tough and cannot be compressed. Once planted the seed will start to expand and can be compressed.

- Uniform expansion in all directions with no resistance
- Support by allowing space for growth

2. Vayu = unidirectional movement

Now seed starts to bulge in one direction.

- Unilateral expansion
- Propulsion
- Movement in a single direction

3. Agni/Tejas = conversion

With the sudden breaking of foliage and the stem coming out due to a change of temperature (thermogenesis).

- Conversion
- Transformation

4. Apas/Jala = cohesion

No change in temperature yet growth continues.

- Growing
- Increasing, unit by unit

5. Prthivi = solidification

Liquid material gets solidity in particular place and gives a specific form.

- Shape
- Size
- solidity

Conclusion

By creating a space (Akasha) - then establishing a direction (Vayu) – then through heat a new transformation process is created (Agni) - then growth takes place (Jala) - until it takes a final solid form (Prthivi).

The Five Great Elements of States of Matter (Pancha Mahabhutani)				
Tanmatras	Sound (Śabda)	Touch (Sparśa)	Sight (Rūpa)	Taste (Rasa)	Smell (Gandha)
Mahabhutani	Ether (Akāśa)	Wind (Vāyu)	Fire (Agni)	Water (Apas)	Earth (Pṛthivi)
Jnanendriyani	Ears	Skin	Eyes	Tongue	Nose
Karmendriyani	Mouth (Expression)	Hands (Grasping)	Feet (Motion)	Urino-genital (Emission)	Anus (Elimination)
State of Matter	Field	Gaseous	Transformative / Radiant	Humidity / Liquidity	Density
Attribute	Space	Movement	Heat	Cohesion	Solidity
Concepts	Connection, communication unity	Movement, direction, penetration	Transformation light, perception	Cohesion, binding, holding	Density, solidity, stability
Prānas	Prāna (Reception)	Udāna (Expression)	Samāna (Balance)	Vyāna (Circulation)	Apāna (Elimination)
Tissues Nourished by the Elements	The five senses and the mind	Bone (Asthi)	Digestive bile (Agni), Blood (Rakta)	Plasma (Rasa), Fat (Meda), Nerves (Majja), Fertility (Shukra)	Muscle (Mamsa)

Chapter Three Study Questions

1. What are the Gurvadi Gunah?

2. Where do the 20 Gunas or attributes come from?

3. Rajas Guna relates to which of the 20 attributes?

4. Why are the 20 Gunas are central to understanding Ayurvedic therapeutics?

5. Which areas of Ayurveda do we use the Gurvadi Gunas?

6. Which Guna is oily?

7. Which Guna is penetrating?

8. Which Guna is liquid?

9. Which Guna is dry?

10. Which Guna is dull?

CHAPTER FOUR
THE TRIDOSHA THEORY

Often Ayurveda is said to rest on the *Tridosha* theory. What does this term mean and what role does it play in Ayurvedic medicine? The ancient Rishi's that developed Ayurveda observed nature closely for hundreds of years. The outcome of their observations was that the physical universe is composed of four primary states of matter – a solid state of matter; a liquid state of matter; matter in a state of transformation; and matter in movement. These four states of matter exist in a fifth state, a field or space. This is called the *Pancha Maha Bhutani*, or five great states of matter. This concept was explained in the Samkhya Darshana and the previous chapter.

The ancients also observed that some principle controls, or manages, these five different states of matter. According to their observation three principles, or Dosha (Dosha), perform this function. According to the Samkhya Darshana these principles manifest at the level of the Tanmatras or subtle matter, or matter as energy. The ancient text describe the Dosha as coming from the life-force or Prana. The Dosha are actually three forms of Prana that exist to manage the five states of matter in living organisms.

The Tridosha theory is that idea which states that matter is governed by three managers. These managers, or Dosha, are intelligent because they come from Prana - the intelligent principle of energy in the universe. Also, as stated in Samkhya Darshana everything that exists in the manifestation comes from pure consciousness, Atman, or Purusha and therefore is intelligent.

These principles are biological forces and can be seen, or their actions can be observed, by anyone. Knowing that living organisms are controlled by intelligent managers that are either observable, or their actions are observable, is called the *'Tridosha'* theory and forms the basis of the Ayurvedic system.

It is important to understand that the Dosha can be used in several different ways in Ayurveda. For example, the three Doshas have physiological functions, so are therefore part of Anatomy and Physiology. The Doshas are also used to determine the constitution or *Prakriti* of any person. They are also used in pathology to determine the causes and types of diseases. The three Doshas are also used in relation to time and the movement of time as per the delineations of the day, or year. Hence, we see that the concept of three Dosha is actually quite vast and needs to be approached in a methodical manner to avoid confusion.

Ayurveda has become vulgarized through time and its introduction to the Western cultures. One of the primary distinctions between Ayurvedic Medicine and Ayurvedic

Wellness is the incorrect use of the Tridosha theory. In Wellness the Dosha are used very little. If they are used it is to offer an oil massage or treatment according to the dominate Dosha - or Prakriti. Usually, Wellness Ayurveda does not go beyond the idea of individual constitutions - Prakriti. Wellness focuses more on the symptomatic side of using Indian herbs and oils to present the illusion of Ayurvedic medicine, when in fact it is not.

Ayurvedic Medicine uses the Dosha to understand the structures of the body (anatomy), the functions of the body (physiology), the cause of disease (aetiology), the manifesting of symptoms (symptomatology), diagnosis, the manifestation of disease (pathogenesis), and the classification of disease. Additionally, the cycles of day and night, the cycles of the seasons, and the cycles of human age, are all controlled by Dosha. The correct use of Dosha in each of these instances required study, correct instruction and an intelligent application. If this is not done the Tridosha theory will not create health - it will create disease.

In order to understand the Dosha correctly we should first begin to understand their role in anatomy and physiology as this is their primary function.

Overview of the Dosha

The word *Dosha* means "that which is stained" or "that which has a fault". In other words, the meaning of *Dosha* has a basically negative connotation. Why would something that is responsible to maintain life be given a title that is basically negative?

First it is important to understand that Ayurvedic Tridosha theory and anatomy / physiology is based on the concept of "functioning". Modern anatomy and physiology is based on the "location" of things; therefore, there are no managers or Dosha. Hence, Ayurveda views the body more through systems and their relations. Whereas modern medicine views the body through form and structure.

Form of Medicine	Primary Concept:	Creates:	Results in:
Ayurvedic Medicine	Function	Network of systems	Interrelations
Modern Medicine	Location	Individual structures	Separate forms

Therefore, when we understand that Dosha function is at the heart of Ayurvedic anatomy and physiology we begin to see the challenges faced by these managers. The Doshas begin working prior to birth. The stop working at death. This means that from pre-birth to death the Doshas are functioning - in other words, working non-stop. No vacations, no rest. If a person follows an Ayurvedic lifestyle the Doshas can manage to maintain health. However, if a person begins to work in excess, travel in excess, eat or drink in excess, do anything in excess - or not do anything - then Dosha have a very, very hard time to do their job. Their work is so difficult that the Caraka Samhita says:

"The three Doshas, Vata, Pitta and Kapha are the cause of all pathology in the physical body. The Gunas, Raja and Tamas are the cause of all pathology in the mind."
CS.SU.1.57

These are some of the reasons why Ayurveda uses the term "Dosha" to indicate the managers of the five states of matter:
1. they are the cause of pathology (disease)
2. they never get a rest
3. they are directly affected by our lifestyle and habits
4. they are influenced by the movement of time (day/night, seasons and age)
5. they are influenced by the environment
6. they are influenced by the mind

In fact the three Dosha have a difficult vocation to maintain health in any individual. In order to do this they first need to do their job correctly and secondary they need to co-operate with the other two Dosha. They need to maintain the internal environment and respond correctly to changes in the external environment. They need to constantly adapt to the aging process of an individual and either the increase or decrease of food and exercise. Any failure of these multiple activities results in the beginning of pathology.

Additional, the Dosha are modified by the psychological states that result from the three Maha Guna - Sattva, Rajas, Tamas. Any mental shock will not only disrupt the three Gunas in the mind, it will also disrupt the three Dosha function in the body. Thus, the three Dosha need to co-ordinate both the physical manifestations of body / environment and the mental / psychological states.

- According to Ayurveda there are three primary Doshas in the body (Tridosha).
- They are the primary forces behind all physiological functions.
- They produce and maintain the body structure.
- They are also causative factors in disease pathology.
- Ayurveda is a functional system of medicine that uses managers (Dosha).
- Systems need managers (Dosha) to control the functions within them.
- Tridosha theory is one of the most important concepts in Ayurveda.

The basic idea of Ayurvedic medicine is that the body is in constant movement and change due to the above mentioned factors (environment, food, habits, psychology, etc.). This is why Ayurveda is fundamentally a "functional system of medicine". Below we find the primary "functions" of the Tridosha.
- Vata governs all Dosha coordination, movement in general, thus controls all nervous functions and mobility; anything that moves in the body does so due to Vata, including the two other Dosha.

- Pitta governs transformation, thus is responsible for all chemical and metabolic functions, giving heat to the body and the ability to digest, assimilate and transform things.

- Kapha relates to cohesion and thus provides structure, support, stability, and lubrication to the body.

These Dosha carry out these functions through a network of channels or systems. They are responsible for the creation and maintenance of all structure (tissues) in the body.

- Vata manages Wind (Vayu) and Ether (Akasha) elements. It makes them work together to produce all kinds of movements in the body. Movement needs space to define limits. Just think of the lungs. The relationship between space (the changing volume of the lungs) creates a movement of air.

- Pitta manages Fire (Agni) and Water (Jala) elements. These manifest as hot liquids like bile and blood.

- Kapha manages Water (Jala) and Earth (Prthivi). These elements allow Kapha to create its protective substances, like mucous, lymph, cerebrospinal fluid, synovial fluid, as well as all soft tissues in general.

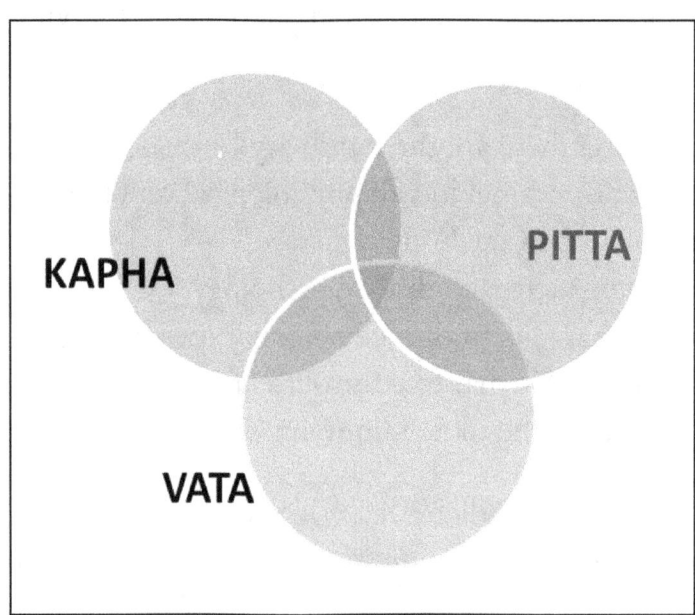

The Dosha as part of Anatomy

The Indian methodology to understand anything is through the twenty attributes or twenty Gunas that was explained in the last chapter. In Ayurveda whenever we want to understand something we observe what attributes are dominate. We use this method in all the different applications of Ayurveda. One of the key concepts in Ayurveda is the Tridosha theory and it is necessary to learn by heart the attributes that are associated with them. These twenty attributes are used throughout all aspects of Ayurvedic medicine and should be memorized.

The main textbook we will use for the study of Anatomy and Physiology is the Ashtanga Hrdayam. In this book Vagbhata gives an easier description of Anatomy and Physiology than both Caraka and Susruta. He begins with the twenty qualities of the three Dosha.

Qualities of the Doshas

Vata

Tridosalaksana—(properties of the three doṣas)—

तत्र रूक्षो लघुः शीतः खरः सूक्ष्मश्चलोऽनिलः ।

Rūkṣa (dryness), laghu (light in weight), śīta (coldness), khara (roughness), sūkṣma (subtleness) and cala (movement) are the properties of Anila (vāta).

Pitta

पित्तं सस्नेहतीक्ष्णोष्णं लघु विस्रं सरं द्रवम् ॥११॥

Sasneha (slight unctousness), tīkṣṇa (penetrating deep), uṣṇa (hot, heat producing), laghu (light in weight), visra (bad smell), sara (free flowing) and drava (liquidity) are the properties of Pitta.

Kapha

स्निग्धः शीतो गुरुमन्दः श्लक्ष्णो मृत्स्नः स्थिरः कफः ।

Snigdha (unctousness), śīta (cold, producing coldness), guru (heavy), manda (slow in action), slakṣṇa (smooth), mṛtsna (slimy) and sthira (stable/static) are the properties of kapha.

What is obvious by these sutras is that **Vata Dosha** shows the following attributes in the following order:

- Dry, light, cold, rough, subtle and movement.

It is important to understand that only Vata has *Chala Guna* or mobility. Vata is the only Dosha that can move and is responsible to move the other two Doshas. Unfortunately, some Western teachers have indicated that Pitta is also mobile - this is totally wrong and causes a number of problems in the clinical application of Ayurvedic medicine.

Note that even though Vata is the only Dosha that can move, mobility is the last of the attributes indicated. The first and most important is dryness followed by lightness. Then we see that coldness, roughness and subtlety are next, ending with movement. These attributes need to be memorized in this order as they are mandatory for correct diagnosis and treatment of many disorders.

In these sutras **Pitta Dosha** shows the following attributes in the following order:

- Slightly oily, penetrating, hot, light, malodorous, spreading and liquid.

It is important to understand that only Pitta has heat due to the fire element (Agni bhuta). Only Pitta keep the body warm and only Pitta can transform food, air, liquids due to the fire element it manages. Pitta is not mobile (chala Guna) but it has an attribute associated with fire that is *Sara Guna* – spreading. This means that Pitta can invade an area or zone of the body through the burning, spreading action of fire.

Note however that the oily attribute is listed as first with the penetrating attribute as second. This indicates that Pitta can quickly penetrate into deep levels of the body while keeping the tissues hydrated (the slightly oily Guna hydrates and lubricates). So unlike Vata that - due to its subtle attributes - can penetrate and dry out the tissues, Pitta can maintain and hydrate the tissues; or it can penetrate them and burn them up.

In these sutras **Kapha Dosha** shows the following attributes in the following order:

- Oily, coolness, heavy, slow, smooth, slimy and static.

Only Kapha provides static stability. The other two Dosha are both light in attributes. This means that Kapha is the only Dosha that can support and maintain the body. Note however that it is the oily attribute that is listed first. This gives top importance to the lubricating qualities of Kapha. Combined with smooth and slimy Gunas Kapha is able to counter the light, dry and hot attributes of Vata and Pitta.

Vata – Wind – That Which Moves Things – Movement
- dry (rūkśa), light (laghu), cold (śīta), rough (khara), subtle (sūksma), mobile (cala)
- Sanskrit root 'va' = to blow, flow, direct or command
- Vata is the coldest, Kapha is cool.
- Vata is the moving force behind Pitta and Kapha—who are lame without Vata
- Vata is the prime force of the nervous system
- Governs sensory and mental balance, sensory and motor coordination
- Gives mental adaptability and comprehension
- Vata coordinates the whole body and the other Doshas
- Supported or contained by Ether—resides in empty spaces in the body, colon, pores in bones.

Pitta – Bile – That Which Digests Things – Transformation
- little oily (sasneha), sharp/penetrating (tīksna), hot (usna), light (laghu), bad smell (visra), flowing/liquid (sara/drava)
- Sanskrit root 'tap' = to heat, cook, transform.
- Pitta is hot.
- Responsible for all chemical and metabolic functions in the body.
- Governs our digestion, capacity to perceive reality and understand things as they are.
- Supported by Water element it exists mainly in an acid form (digestive juices, blood).

Kapha – Phlegm – Which Holds Things Together – Cohesion
- wet (snigdha), cold (śīta), heavy (guru), slow (manda), smooth (slaksna), slimy (mrtsna), static (sthira).
- The word Kapha is derived from the Sanskrit root 'Slish' which means to bind or hold together.
- Kapha is cool, Vata is cold.
- Gives nourishment, substance, support—makes up the bulk of bodily tissues.
- Provides lubrication for all tissues.
- Kapha serves as a vehicle, or substratum for Vata and Pitta.
- Supported/contained in the medium of Earth – resides in skin, tissue linings and muscles.

Shared Qualities

Each of the Doshas shares one major quality and is opposite in two others:-
- LIGHT – Vata and Pitta share light/subtle qualities which provide perception and penetration.
- COLD – Both Vata and Kapha reduce bodily heat. Vata disperses heat, Kapha

conserves it in the tissues.
- MOIST – Pitta and Kapha both supply bodily fluids: Pitta (liquefying / heating force) as in blood and its circulation. Kapha (oily / nurturing) as in plasma which nourishes entire body including the blood.

Sites of the Doshas

Vata – colon, thighs, hips, ears, bones, skin, ears, brain
- Colon is the main site of liquid and nutrient absorption
- Thighs and hips are the main site of musculoskeletal movement in the body.
- Sense organs of hearing and touch as per ether and air elements correspondence with Vata.

Pitta – small intestine, stomach, sweat, sebaceous glands, blood, lymph, eyes.
- Small intestine is the main site of the digestive fire or Agni.
- Stomach is the site of the digestive acids that are a secondary site of Agni.
- Sweat and sebaceous glands hold and release heat.
- Blood holds heat and color.
- Sense organ of sight as pertaining to the element fire and perception.

Kapha – stomach, chest, throat, head, pancreas, sides, lymph, fat, nose, tongue and reproductive system
- Chest, lungs, throat, head, sinuses and nasal passages produce phlegm / Kapha.
- Mouth and tongue also produce saliva (a Kapha fluid).
- Fat tissue stores Snigdha and nutrients.
- Abdominal cavity is surrounded by peritoneal fluid.
- Reproductive system holds fluid such as sperm and ovum.
- Sense organs of taste and smell as per water and earth elements.

Sites of the Doshas According to Ashtanga Hrdayam

Doṣasthāna—(*seats of doṣas*) :—

पक्वाशयकटीसक्थिश्रोत्रास्थिस्पर्शनेन्द्रियम् ।
स्थानं वातस्य, तत्रापि पक्वाधानं विशेषतः ॥ १ ॥

Pakvāśaya (large intestine), waist, thigh, ear, bone and the organ of touch (skin) are the seats of vāta, especially, so the pakvādhāna (large intestine). 1.

नाभिरामाशयः स्वेदो लसीका रुधिरं रसः ।
दृक् स्पर्शनं च पित्तस्य, नाभिरत्र विशेषतः ॥ २ ॥

Nābhi (umbilicus), āmāśaya (stomach and small intestine), sweat, lasīka (lymph), blood, rasa (plasma), eye, and the organ of touch (skin), are the seats of pitta, especially so the nābhi (region around the umbilicus). 2.

उरः कण्ठशिरः क्लोमपर्वाण्यामाशयो रसः ।
मेदो घ्राणं च जिह्वा च कफस्य, सुतरामुरः ॥ ३ ॥

Chest, throat, head, kloma (pancreas ?), bony joints, āmāśaya (stomach and small intestine), rasa (plasma), fat, nose and tongue are the seats of kapha, especially so the chest. 3.

The Doshas exist everywhere in the body as they control function. However, Ayurveda considers that each Dosha has a "home" or primary site where it accumulates. This is called the "sthana". It can also be called the mula sthana or "root site" or primary site. The primary sites of the Doshas (*mulasthana*) are very important since these are where Doshas will congregate when they start to accumulate.

- Vata's primary site is the colon
- Pitta's primary site is the small intestine
- Kapha's primary site is the stomach

It is also possible to make a correlation between the location of the five states of matter and three doshas in the body. The following chart shows the relationship by location in the body.

Balance Relationships between Elements & Doshas

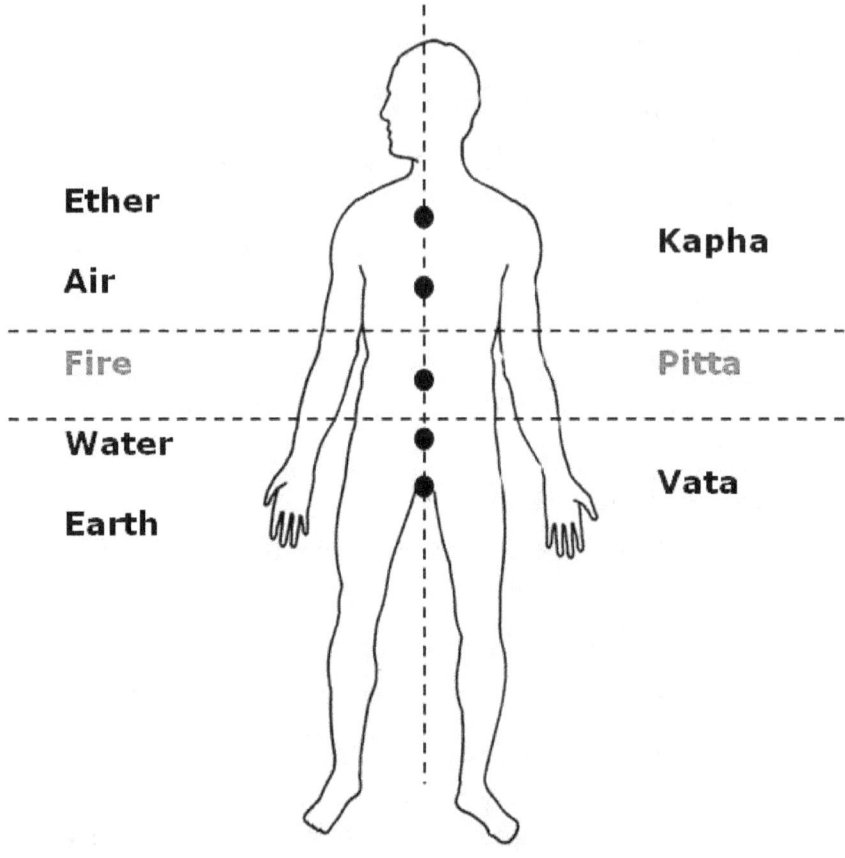

Ether & Air allows Kapha space to move.
Fire allows both Kapha & Vata heat in
which to function.
Water & Earth allows stability for Vata.

As the chart above indicates the location of the three dosha and the five states of matter are not the same in the body. The five elements have a complementary relationship to the three dosha. Note that heavy earth and water are in the Vata zone and light either and wind (air) are in the Kapha zone. This acts to balance out the dosha. For example, we would not be able to breathe if either and air where not there to create "space" in the zone of heavy, lubricating Kapha. Likewise, Vata would not be able to stay in one place if there was not earth and water to anchor Vata down to the ground.

The classical description of anatomy in Ayurveda is the following sutra:

Dosā-dhātū-malā mūlam sadā dehasya tam calah |
Asthanga Hrdayam, Sutrasthana, 11.1

Here is the English translation and explanation of this sutra:

Dehasya mūlam—(chief constituents of the body) :--

दोषधातुमला मूलं सदा देहस्य

Doṣās, Dhātūs (tissues) and malas (waste products) are the roots (causes, chief constituents, supports), of the body always (throughout the span of life.) 1.

Notes :--Doṣās are of two kinds, (a). Śarīra (somatic) viz, vāta, pitta and kapha, (b). mānasa (psychic) viz, rajas and tamas. Dhātus (tissues) are seven viz, rasa (plasma), rakta (blood), mamsa (muscle), medas (fat), asthi (bone), majja (bone marrow) and śukra (semen–the reproductive tissue in the males and its counter part ārtava (ovum) in females). Ojas the essence of the dhātus is counted as the eighth dhātu. In addition, there are some upadhātus (secondary tissues) such as lasīkā (lymph), stanya (breast milk), kaṇḍarā (tendons) sira dhamanī (veins and arteries), vasā (muscle fat), twak (skin), snāyu (nerves), taruṇāsthi (cartillages) etc; malās (waste products) are puriṣa (feaces), mūtra (urine), sweda (sweat), kha-mala (dhātu mala-waste products of tissues). excretions of the eyes, nose, ears, of the small and big channels, etc. keśa-roma (hair on the head and body), nakha (nails) etc.

All these are present in the human body always throughout life. So long as they are normal (in their quantity, qualities and function) they maintain the health of the person and when they become abnormal, they become causes of diseases. This will be described in this chapter and also the next.

Ayurveda views nature as its primary teacher. Thus, the idea of a 'root' is very important because a root nourishes and supports the plant. Without roots the plant cannot exist. Therefore, *Dosha, Dhatu, Mala* is an important concept in Ayurveda as they form the 'root' or main support for the human body.

We will study Dhatu (tissues) and Malas (waste products) in other lessons. So let us go onward to the function of dosha now that we have seen their attributes and physical locations in the body.

The Dosha as part of Physiology

The definition of physiology is: "*Physiology is the science of the functioning of living systems. In physiology, the scientific method is applied to determine how organisms, organ systems, organs, cells and biomolecules carry out the chemical or physical function that they have in a living system.*"

In Ayurveda physiology is the study of how doshas function. Therefore, we begin by the understanding that all functions in the body, on all levels, are carried out by dosha. So it will not matter if we if speak of a muscle cell or of a whole muscle such as the triceps. This is because we are concerned with FUNCTION and not structure when speaking about dosha. When we study the Dahtu then this will change because that will be the study of structure. So as long as the subject is dosha their functions will apply on all levels of the body. Here is a description of their main functions:

Vata – Responsible for all physiological and organic processes in general.
- Governs the other two Doshas
- It is the most important as it is the root of the Doshas, tissues and waste materials.
- In its natural state it sustains effort/energy, breathing, movement, discharge of impulses, equilibrium of tissues (homeostasis), coordination of the senses.
- Imbalances of Vata are thus usually more severe and effect the entire body.

Pitta – Governs light and heat in the body.
- Governs digestion, heat, visual perception, hunger, thirst, luster, complexion, and softness of the body.
- It involves the combustion of materials that give warmth and color.
- It is involved in all transformative processes.

Kapha – Material substratum/support for the other two Doshas.
- Gives stability, lubrication, holding together of the joints.
- Conserving and restraining force on other two Doshas and their active and consuming nature.
- Without Kapha, Vata and Pitta would disperse and disintegrate the body.
- Lubricates the mucus membranes and joints and cushions the entire body.

The classics are a little different in their description. Again is best to use the Asthanga Hrdayam to understand the Dosha function in physiology. As indicated earlier in this book the Asthanga is more modern syntheses of the older texts. The other reason is that the information in the Asthanga works well clinically even today. Hence, it is a good place to start from when trying to understand Ayurvedic physiology.

In terms of function Vata is the most important dosha because it coordinates the other doshas and animates them through Cala Guna, or movement. Vata is also the functional link between the mind and body. From a Yogic point of view (Yoga Darshana) this is done through the second sheath, or *pranamayakosha*. This Kosha, or sheath, mediates between the body (*anamayakosha*) and the psychology (*manomayakosha*). From a more mechanical point of view of pure Ayurvedic anatomy this communication between mind and body happens through two channels or *Srota* called the *pranavhasrota* and the *manovahasrota*. Hence, due to Vata's capacity to link the psychology with the physiology it establishes itself as the dominant dosha.

The classic texts state that both Pitta and Kapha are "lame" without Vata. This means that Vata is the animating force behind both Pitta and Kapha. This is why I insist in this textbook that only Vata Dosha has Cala Guna and can move. Neither Pitta nor Kapha can move without Vata. This is one of the secrets in clinical practice.

Functions of the Doshas

Prakṛta doṣa karma--(*functions of normal doṣas*) :--

तं चलः ।

उत्साहोच्छ्वासनिश्वासचेष्टावेगप्रवर्तनैः ॥ १ ॥

सम्यग्गत्या च धातूनामक्षाणां पाटवेन च ।

अनुगृह्णात्यविकृतः, पित्तं पक्त्यूष्मदर्शनैः ॥ २ ॥

क्षुत्तृड्रुचिप्रभामेधाधीशौर्यतनुमार्दवैः ।

श्लेष्मा स्थिरत्वस्निग्धत्वसन्धिबन्धक्षमादिभिः ॥ ३ ॥

Out of them cala (vāta), in its normal state, protects the body bestowing enthusiasm (eagerness, desire), expiration and inspiration, all activities (of the body, mind and speech), initiation (and also execution) of the urges (of faeces, urine etc.), maintainence of the dhātus (tissues) in their normalcy and proper functioning of the sense organs.

Pitta, in its normal state attends to digestion, maintainence of body temperature, vision, production of hunger, thirst, appetite, complexion, intellegence, courage, valour, and softness (suppleness) of the body.

Śleṣman (kapha) confers stability, lubrication, compactness (firmness) of the joints, forbearance (capacity to withstand or withhold emotions, strain etc.) and such others. 1½–3.

Notes :--The above are only the chief functions, they also attend to many others also.

This sutra is one of the most important in the Ashtanga Hrdayam.

Note the first indication of Vata. "In its normal state it protects the body and bestows enthusiasm...."

By function Vata is the most important of all dosha. It protects us and gives us the desire to live. It gives the interest (enthusiasm) to create, to live, to experience this wonderful universe. Read the above sutra carefully and you will see that the control of Vata is the key to health and happiness in this incarnation. Both Pitta and Kapha support and aid Vata. They are equally important in their own way. However, once in a clinical environment the key to success with most patients will be a correct understanding of this sutra. If Vata Dosha functions correctly everything becomes much easier in treatments – no matter what therapy is used.

Table Showing Functions of the Three Doshas

Vata Movement	Pitta Transformation	Kapha Cohesion
Movement Circulation Respiration Elimination Reproductive cycles All physiological and organic processes in general Governs Pitta and Kapha Effort Discharge of impulses Equilibrium of tissues Coordination of senses Enthusiasm Mental coordination Mental adaptability	Controls light and heat in the body Digestion Metabolism Hunger Thirst Combustion of materials that give warmth and colour Lustre Complexion Softness of the body Visual perception Mental perception Understanding Courage	Material substratum for the other two Doshas Stability to the body Lubricates the mucus membranes and joints Holding together of the joints Cushions the entire body Acts to conserve and restrain the other two Doshas Reproductive fertility Physical endurance Patience Compassion Nurturing

- When something needs to be moved – Vata activates.
- When something needs to be transformed – Pitta activates.
- When something needs to be built, lubricated or protected – Kapha activates.

At all other times, the Doshas rest and await their next command. They are only active when needed. Note that many aspects of Dosha function, like homeostasis, breathing, heart beating, require a continuous effort of the Doshas; whereas other functions such as elimination or talking do not.

Chapter Four Study Questions

1. How would you accurately define the Doshas?

2. Are Doshas always functioning?

3. Why is Vata the most important Dosha generally?

4. What is the most important Guna of Vata Dosha?

5. What Gunas are shared by Pitta and Kapha?

6. Why are the mulasthana (main sights or 'seats' of the Doshas) so important?

7. Are Vata and Kapha are equally cold?

8. How do Doshas help us understand anatomy and physiology?

9. What is the mulasthana of Pitta?

10. What is Kapha Dosha?

CHAPTER FIVE
THE SUB DOSHA IN ANATOMY & PHYSIOLOGY

Each of the three doshas has a subdivision of five aspects, each aspect controlling a function or system of the body. The sub dosha offers a precision of the global dosha function. For example: as Vata controls movement the five forms of Vata will control five different kinds of movement; the five Pittas five different forms of transformation, and the five Kapha five forms of lubrication. The five sub doshas exist because of the five Tanmatras that manifest after Manas and before the five elements or states of matter. Because there are five Tanmatras there cannot be four or six sub doshas. Just as there cannot be a sixth category of matter, there cannot be a sixth sub division of the dosha.

Vata -In general Vata controls all movement in the body and mind, it is the principal of movement in nature and in the body. Hence, it relates directly to the nervous system which controls all movement. It relates to the systems of circulation, respiration, muscular movement, motor function, the five senses, evacuation, lactation, menstruation, sexual function, and sweating. Vata is directly related to the bones and bone structure. Together with Pitta it controls the hormonal function. The other two doshas are inert without Vata. It coordinates all functions of the body through itself and the other two doshas. The five subdivisions control the various aspects of this general description.

Prana vayu - Controls inhalation, the other four vayus (Vata), the five senses, thinking, overall health, and proper growth. Pervading the head and centered in the brain Prana moves downward to the chest and throat. It governs inhalation and swallowing, and sneezing. It governs the intake of impressions through the five senses that are received through the five senses.
Indications of Imbalance - loss of senses, anxiety and worry, insomnia, dryness, emaciation, disease in general

Udana vayu - Controls exhalation, speech, and the upward movements in the body, growth as a child. Udana is located in the chest and centered in the throat and governs exhalation. It has primarily an upward movement and brings the air up and out of the body in exhalation. Udana also brings our enthusiasm up and outwards into our endeavors. It causes our mind, will and consciousness to ascend.

Indications of Imbalance - problems of speech and the throat, weakness of will, general fatigue, lack of enthusiasm

Samana vayu - Controls the movement of the digestive system, the solar plexus and balances the prana and apana vayus. It is centered in the small intestine and governs the process of digestion and assimilation of nutrients. Samana is the predominant Vata in the internal organs including the liver, spleen, pancreas, stomach, and upper portion of the colon. It mainly has an equalizing or balancing action and balances the higher and lower portions of the body. Samana works as a centripetal ("center-seeking") force directing substances in the body to the digestive area for transformation. Vyana then transports the nutrients away from the digestive organs through its centrifugal ("center-fleeing") action. Together Samana and Vyana form an important polarity.

Indications of Imbalance - upset digestion, indigestion, diarrhea, malabsorption of nutrients, internal dryness.

Vyana vayu - Pervades the entire body as the nervous system, yet it also controls heart function and circulation of the blood. It is centered in the heart and distributed throughout the entire body. It governs the movement of the joints and muscles (musculoskeletal system). Vyana's action is primarily in the legs and arms, the main sites of movement in the body. It has an important role at night to circulate around the body and collect waste material from the normal metabolism of tissues. This waste is collected by Vyana and given to Samana who carries it to the digestive organs for removal. Vyana transports the nutrients away from the digestive organs through its centrifugal ("center-fleeing") action in order to nourish all the tissues. Together with Samana it forms an important polarity.

Indications of Imbalance - arthritis, nervousness, poor circulation, poor motor reflexes, problems of the joints, bone disorders, nervous disorders.

Apana vayu- Controls elimination, sexual function, menstruation, downward movements in the body, elimination of wastes and disease in general. Apana is centered in the colon and governs all downward moving impulses of elimination, urination, menstruation, parturition and orgasm. It also governs the absorption of water and micronutrients in the colon and allows the full absorption of nutrients from our food. Apana supports and controls all the other forms of Vata because it is the only form of Vata that does not move constantly. Apana only moves when needed (i.e., urination, etc.). By not moving it creates a stable platform for the other forms of Vata. This is why the large intestine is Vata's main site or Mulasthana. Derangements of Apana are implicated in most Vata disorders. Therefore, the treatment of Apana is one of the first considerations in the treatment of Vata.

Indications of Imbalance - constipation, menstrual problems, dryness, urinary problems, generally all diseases are involved.

The Pancha Vayu (five forms of Vata Dosha)

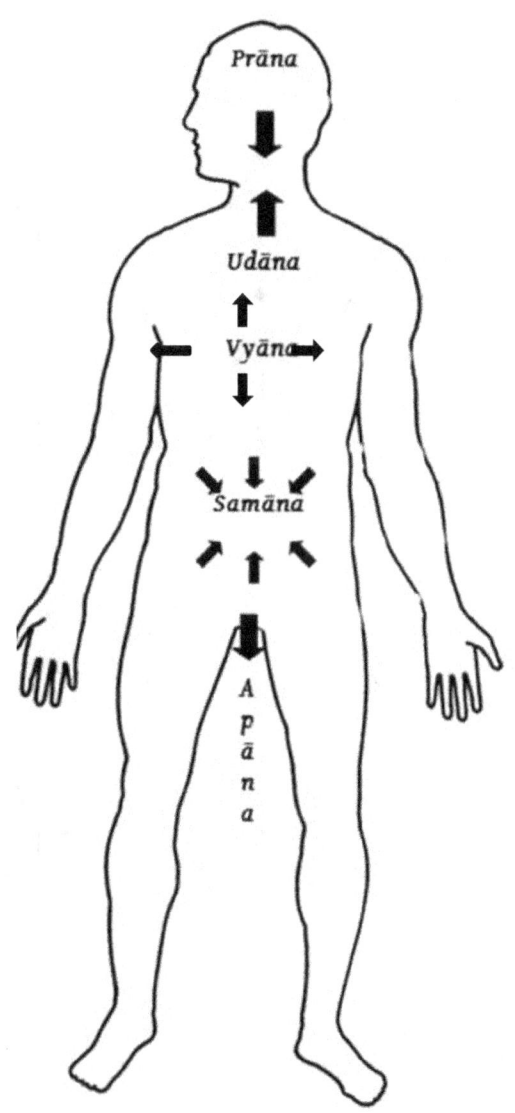

Polarities with the Vayus

First and most important is	Prana & Apana	(in & out)
Next important is	Udana & Apana	(up & down)
Then the last is	Samana &Vyana	(center & outer)

Note that Vata Dosha is the most important in treatments and therefore this information needs to me memorized.

Prāna Vāyu—Primary Air (wind)

Intake of Energy

In & Down

In Breath

RECEPTION

Principle Sites

· **HEAD** - senses and mental functions
· **HEART** - Beating of heart and movement of lungs

Governs

· All other Vayus
· Inhalation
· Swallowing
· Sneezing
· Spitting
· Mind (Thoughts, Emotions, Feelings, Knowledge)
· Heart
· Consciousness
· Energy
· Coordination
· Adaptability
· Directs other Vayus

Gives

· Inspiration
· Vitality
· Connects us with outside

Actions

· Right receptivity
· Openness to Divine
· Balanced psychology
· Positive Attitude
· Controls the 5 senses

Development

· Pranayama
· Meditation
· Mantra

Disturbed

· Disorders of the mind
· Disorders of the senses
· Nervous disorders
· All diseases involve some impairment of Prana Vayu.

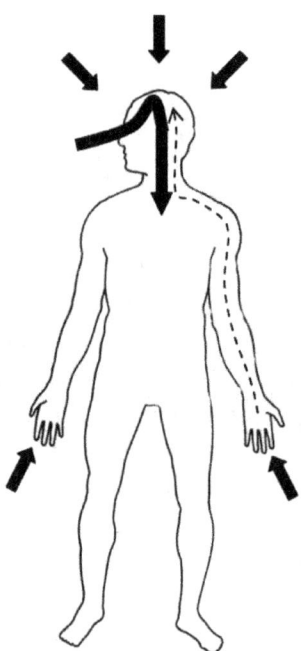

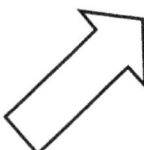

Primary Life Force

Udāna Vāyu—Upward Moving Air (wind)

Output of Energy

Up & Out

Ultimate Result of Nutrition

OUTPUT

Principle Sites

· **THROAT** – allows expression & sits in the throat area, but moves from base of spine to head

Governs

· Exhalation
· Speech
· Memory
· Strength
· Will
· Effort
· Belching

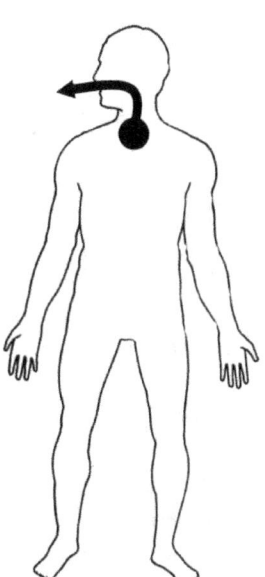

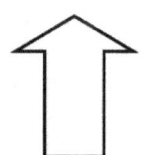

Evolution
of Consciousness
Ascent
of the Life Force

Gives

· Aspiration—moves soul (Jiva) upwards to higher states of consciousness
· Deeper discrimination
· Motivation
· Enthusiasm
· Creative use of Energy
· Power to transcend outer world
· Psychic powers
· Higher values
· Kundalini is refined Udana
· At death moves us up to subtle worlds as per will/karma

Actions

· Speech
· Creativity
· Expression
· Self expression

Development

· Pranayama
· Yoga asana
· Mantra

Disturbed

· Cough
· Belching
· Vomiting
· Suppressing the urge to belch, burp, vomit or sneeze increases udana and makes samana increase too.

Samāna Vāyu—Equalising Air (wind)

Balancing Action

Centripetal Action

ABSORPTION

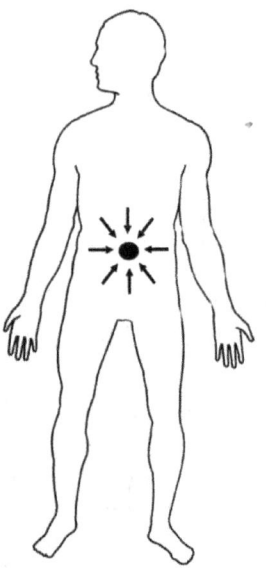
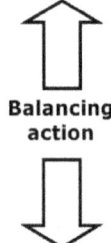

Principle Site

· **NAVEL AREA –** Main Vayu in *Liver, Spleen, Pancreas, Stomach, small intestine*

Governs

· Digestion
· Absorption
· Assimilation
· Manages Pitta & Kapha in digestion

Gives:

· Good digestion
· Balanced Agni
· Stable energy

Actions

· Moves the duodenum, jejunum and ileum.
· Provides stimulus for excretion of digestive juices
· Moves bile from liver, gallbladder and pancreas into the duodenum.

Development

· Pranayama
· Yoga asana

Disturbed

· Lack of Appetite
· Nervous digestion
· Increased/decreased peristalsis
· Bloating
· Colic pain
· Lack of absorption and assimilation

Balancing action

Vyāna Vāyu—Diffusive Air (wind)

Circulation

Centrifugal Action

CIRCULATION

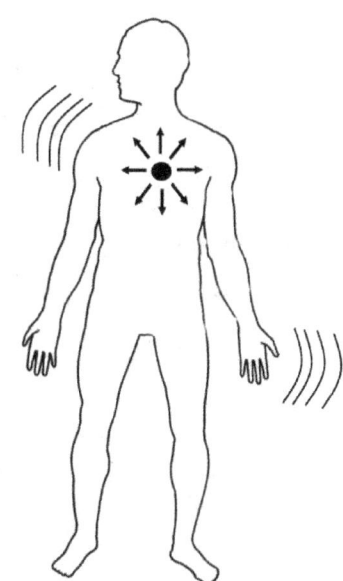

Circulation to the exterior

Principle Sites

· **HEART –** centred in the chest area

· **ALL OVER THE BODY** – vyana is said to live everywhere in the body in the *varuna nadi*

Governs

· Circulation
· Nervous movement
· Muscular movement
· Collecting wastes from Dhatus

Gives:

· Physical capacity
· Right movement
· Stable nervous system

Actions

· Distribution of nutrients
· Circulation of blood
· Nerve movement
· At night time when we sleep, all the vayus rest, except vyana, which collects wastes and deposits them in the organs of elimination.

Development

· Pranayama
· Yoga asana

Disturbed

· Lack of coordination
· Nervous disorders
· Toxic build-up in dhatus
· General pain
· Stiff joints

Apāna Vāyu—Downward Moving Air (wind)

Descending force

Down & Out

Power of disease inherent in body

ELIMINATION

Principle Sites

· **COLON**
· **PELVIC AREA**

Governs

· Elimination
· Menstruation
· Sexual function
· Absorption of liquids
· Final stage of digestion
· allows waste to be removed, menstruation and orgasm.

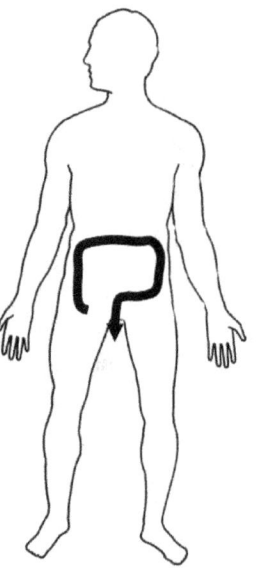

Gives:

· Stability to all Vayus
· Correct nutrient absorption
· Clean tissues
· Stable psychology

Actions

· Does not move except when needed
· Removes waste
· Allows the correct function of all other doshas

Development

· Pranayama
· Yoga asana

Disturbed

· Increase of wastes and toxins
· Disorders of the digestion
· Constipation, diarrhoea
· Loss of strength
· Abnormal discharges
· Irregular Menstruation
· Pain during menstruation.
· Pain during sex
· Premature ejaculation
· Lower backache

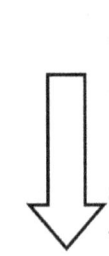

If Vata is high, treat APANA

KEY SUBDOSHA IN TREATMENT

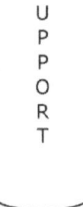

Prana
Udana
Samana
Vyana

S
U
P
P
O
R
T

Pitta - In general Pitta is responsible for all metabolic processes in the body. Pitta is the principal of transformation, on both a mental and physical level. Hence, Pitta helps us to digest thoughts, feelings and food - or transform them into some usable substance. Pitta controls all heat and heat (inflammation) disorders of the body. Together with Vata it controls the hormonal function. Pitta relates to the fiery organs in the body and the blood. It is usually carried by the blood which it controls. Low Pitta will cause the whole metabolism to slow down due to a lack of heat. The five subdivisions control the various aspects of this general description.

Sadhaka Pitta - Controls functions of the heart and the digestion of thoughts and emotions. Sadhaka functions through the nervous system (which includes the brain in Ayurveda) and five senses. It allows one to accomplish goals of the intellect and will. Sadhaka governs the digestion of impressions, ideas or beliefs and our power of discrimination. It is necessary to have Sadhaka to discriminate between the eternal and the transient, the real and the unreal; this is a function of the intellect or Buddhi. When impaired we suffer from lack of clarity, confusion or delusion and become unable to distinguish between our fantasies and reality.
Indications of Imbalance - heart failure, repressed emotions and feelings, excessive anger or unprocessed feelings.

Alochaka Pitta - Controls the ability to see and the digestion of what is seen. It is located in the eyes and is responsible for the reception and digestion of light from the outside. Alochaka has an upward motion that causes the Jivatman to seek light, clarity and understanding. The quality of the Jivatman is visible through the eyes. When impaired we suffer from failure of vision or eye diseases.
Indications of Imbalance - eye problems and difficulties to digest what is seen.

Pachaka Pitta - Controls the digestive system. It is located in the beginning of the small intestine and governs the power of digestion through the control of *Agni*. Pachaka governs the body temperature and helps maintains the overall metabolism. It is the main form of Pitta and supports the other four aspects of Pitta through its heat. It has a discriminating action to recognize the nutritious part of food from the non- nutritious part. Pachaka is responsible for building up our tissues and, with Agni, to destroy pathogens that have entered the body. Pachaka is the first consideration in the treatment of Pitta disorders, as it controls Agni and nutrient transformation in general.
Indications of Imbalance - ulcers, heartburn, cravings, indigestion, food allergies, all digestive problems in general.

Ranjaka Pitta - Controls liver / gall bladder digestion. It is located in the liver, spleen, stomach and small intestine and gives color to the blood, bile and stool. It primarily resides in the liver and controls the *Panchabuta Agnis*. Ranjaka can promote toxins through poor digestion. It colors the secretions of digestive bile and waste materials like urine and feces.

Indications of Imbalance - anger, irritability, hostility, excessive bile, liver disorders, skin problems, toxic blood, anemia.

Bhrajaka Pitta - Controls metabolism of the skin and digestion of light. It is located in the skin and maintains the complexion and skin color. It governs our digestion of sunlight, warmth and heat in general that is absorbed through the skin. Bhrajaka is involved in the process of circulation and governs the heat in the peripheral circulation. Bhrajaka also allows heat to be diffused and dispersed through sweating.

Indications of Imbalance - all skin problems, acne, inflammation of the skin, etc.

Sādhaka Pitta—Power of Discrimination

Mental digestion
and transformation

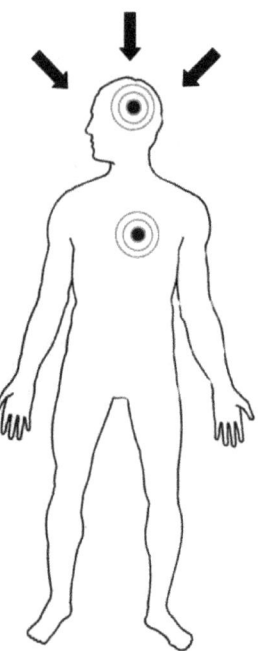

Principle Sites

· **BRAIN**
· **HEART**

Governs

· Mind
· Mental digestion
· Discriminative power
· Buddhi
· Transforms energy from our impressions and life experiences to empower the mind

Gives

· Fire and digestive capacity to mind and senses

Actions

· Accomplish goals of the intellect, intelligence or ego
· Worldly goals of pleasure, wealth and prestige
· Spiritual goal of liberation

Development

· Jnana Yoga
· Passive observation of thoughts
· Meditation

Disturbed

· Lack of clarity
· Confusion
· Lack of discrimination
· Unable to distinguish between fantasies and reality

Alochaka Pitta—Power of Visual Perception

Digestion of light

upward movement

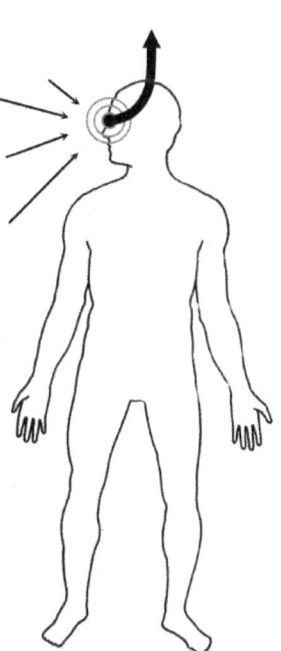

Principle Sites

· **EYES**

Governs

· Reception and digestion of light from the external world
· Feeds the mind by reception of light
· Controls perception

Gives

· Ability to see
· Clearness in eyes means a good digestive power
· Clearness in eyes means deeper intelligence

Actions

· Causes us to seek light, clarity & understanding
· Seeing

Development

· Netra basti
· Looking at nature
· Meditation on light
· Visualization

Disturbed

· Failure of Vision
· Eye diseases

Pācaka Pitta—Power of Digestion

Digestion of food / liquid

balancing action

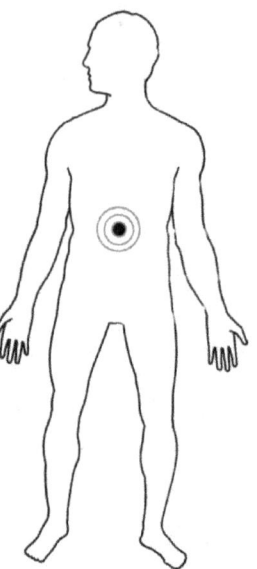

Principle Sites
· **SMALL INTESTINE**
· **LOWER STOMACH**

Governs
· Power of Digestion
· Body temperature
· Jatharagni
· All other forms of Pitta
· Controls enzymes

Gives
· Good digestion
· Good assimilation of nutrients
· Balanced Agni
· Energy
· Body heat

Actions
· Gives bile salts & acids
· Responsible for building up our tissue.
· Helps maintain power of circulation
· Destroys pathogens that enter the body orally.

Development
· Balanced diet
· Fasting
· Yoga asana

Disturbed
· Indigestion
· Ulcers, high agni, Hyperacidity
· poor absorption, lack of body heat, low agni

Sādhaka
Alochaka
Bhrājaka
Rañjaka

S U P P O R T

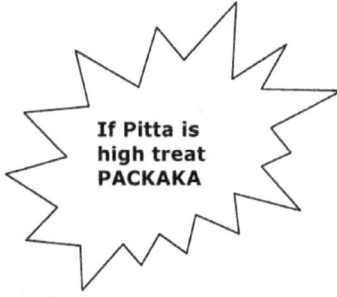

If Pitta is high treat PACKAKA

KEY SUBDOSHA IN TREATMENT

Bhrājaka Pitta—Power of Light Digestion

Digestion of warmth/heat/sunlight

outward moving energy

Principle Sites

· **SKIN**

Governs

· Digestion of external heat absorbed through skin
· Digestion of sunlight
· Complexion
· Luster of skin

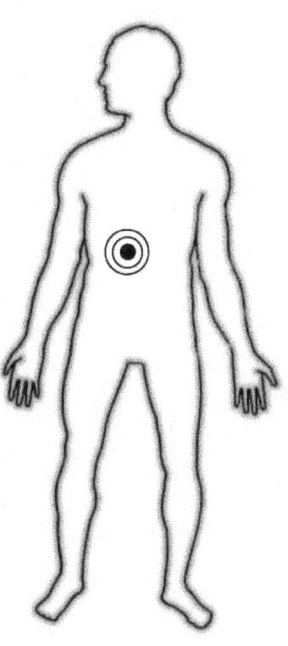

Gives

· Pigmentation
· Skin color
· Skin health

Actions

· Maintains complexion and colour of skin
· Through it we can read the warmth of the body generally
· Through it our heat is diffused and dispersed
· When increased it causes sweating

Development

· Massage
· Exercise
· Svedhana therapies

Disturbed

· Skin rashes
· Skin discolouration

Rañjaka Pitta—Power of Blood Digestion

Digestion of blood

downward moving energy

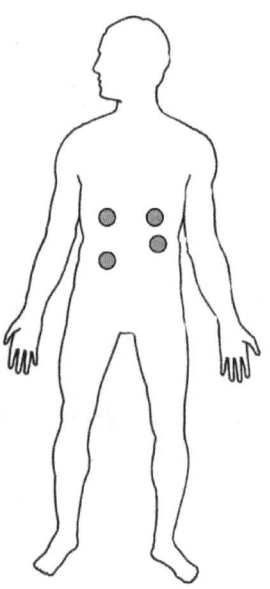

Principle Sites

· **BLOOD**
· **LIVER**
· **SPLEEN**

Governs

· Digestion of blood
· Enzyme functions in the liver and pancreas
· Second stage of digestion or Vipaka

Gives

· Gives color to the blood, bile and stool
· Good digestion
· Skin color

Actions

· Functions as warmth in the blood and circulatory system
· Controls & colors bodily excretions like urine and stool

Development

· Fasting
· Diet
· Personal development to allow emotions
· Hatha Yoga

Disturbed

· Liver disorders
· Blood disorders
· Hepatitis, etc.
· Anaemia
· Yellow eyes

Kapha - In general Kapha is responsible for the stability of our body and mind. Kapha is the principal of cohesion in the body and mind. Kapha mainly exists in the body as plasma, blood, muscle and fat tissues. It provides the lubrication and basic structure of the body. Flexibility and growth are controlled by Kapha. Moisture and fluid retention is maintained by this dosha. The five subdivisions control the various aspects of this general description.

Tarpaka Kapha - Controls fluids in the head, the sinuses and cerebral fluids. It is located in the brain and heart, and supports the cerebrospinal fluid. It gives nourishment and lubrication to the brain and nervous system in general. Tarpaka governs emotional calm and stability, happiness, and memory. It helps to balance both Prana Vayu and Sadhaka Pitta who create dryness and inflammation in the central nervous system.
Indications of Imbalance - sinus problems, headaches, loss of smell

Bodhaka Kapha - Controls taste and the cravings of taste, digestion, and saliva. It is located in the mouth and tongue in the saliva. Like Kledaka, it is part of the first stage of digestion and helps to liquefy the food that is eaten. It governs the sense of taste in general in terms of the artistic and emotional attraction to places, colors and environment. It also has a lubricating role in the nose, eyes, ears and sinuses.
Indications of Imbalance - overeating and cravings for tastes, loss of taste, congestion in the throat, mouth and sinus areas.

Avalambaka Kapha - Controls lubrication and the fluids around the heart, lungs and upper back. It is located in the heart and lungs and lubricates the whole chest area. It relates to the basic plasma (Rasa Dhatu) of the body and helps to produce more unstable Kapha (Asthayi Kapha) through lung and heart action. It creates the mucus membrane of the lungs and it creates stability in our chest and heart. Avalambaka is the reserve of Kapha in general in the body and it supports the function of all other forms of Kapha. Avalambaka causes overweight and most pulmonary disorders, and is the main form of Kapha in the treatment of disease. Its dysfunction is behind most Kapha disorders in the body, hence it is the key subdosha to treat for Kapha.
Indications of Imbalance - congestion in the lungs or heart, stiffness in the back and upper spine, lethargy

Kledaka Kapha - Controls the lubrication of the digestive process, maintains a balance with Pitta, provides internal lubrication. It is located in the stomach and as the mucous lining of the digestive tract. Kledaka is responsible for the liquefaction of food and in the first stage of digestion. It also works in harmony with Pachaka Pitta to protect the mucous lining of the digestive tract from being damaged by the heat of Pachaka Pitta and Agni, the digestive fire.
Indications of Imbalance - bloated stomach, slow or congested digestion, excess mucus in the digestive system

63

Sleshaka Kapha - Controls the lubrication of the joints in the body and aids in all movements. It is located in the joints as the synovial fluid and is responsible for holding the joints together and allowing movement of the body in general. Too much of it causes the joints to swell and too little of it causes dry, cracking joints and difficult movement.

Indications of Imbalance - lose joints, swelling joints, stiff joints, painful movements

Tarpaka Kapha

Lubricates nerves & brain

inward moving action (gives inner happiness)

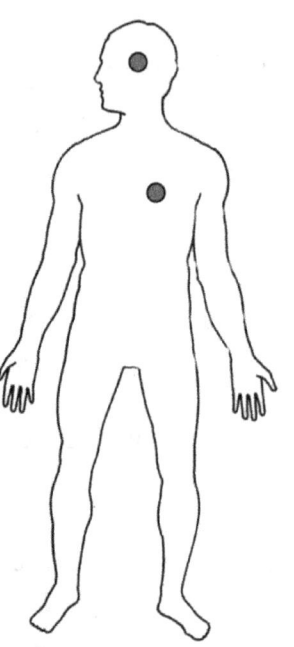

Principle Sites

· **HEAD**
· **HEART**

Governs

· Stability of the mind
· Stability of the nervous system
· Lubrication of heart
· Cerebrospinal fluid

Gives

· Emotional calm, stability and happiness
· Memory capacity
· Stable nerves

Actions

· Maintains the whole body
· Balances Pitta & Vata
· Nourishes and lubricates nerves

Development

· Hatha yoga
· Faith in life
· Meditation
· Bhakti Yoga

Disturbed

· Discontent
· Malaise
· Nervousness
· Insomnia

Bodhaka Kapha

Lubricates mouth / tongue / five senses

upward moving action

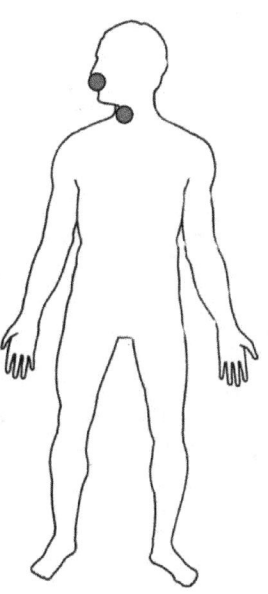

Principle Sites

· **MOUTH**
· **THROAT**

Governs

· Lubrication of heart
· Saliva allowing us to taste
· Pleasure of five senses
· 1st stage of digestion

Gives

· Pleasure
· Stability to senses

Actions

· Lubricates the mouth and beginning of digestive tract
· Controls the senses in the head
· Controls speech

Development

· Fasting
· Moderate Diet
· Hatha Yoga

Disturbed

· Lack of or deranged ability to taste
· sinus disorders
· difficulty with speech or throat

Avalambaka Kapha

Lubricates all dhatus

downward going action (gives support, stability in chest and heart)

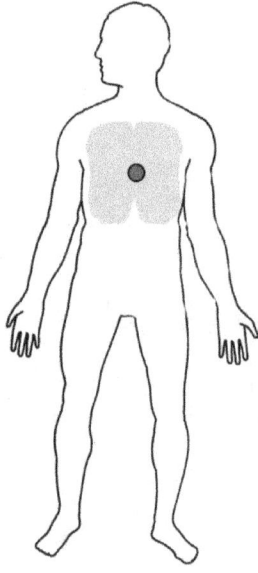

Principle Sites

· **HEART**
· **LUNGS**

Governs

· Lubrication of the heart & lungs
· It is produced by Rasa Dhatu
· It produces Kapha as a waste product
· Overall stability of the body

Gives

· Stability to the chest
· Easy breathing
· Stable heart function

Actions

· Controls Kapha
· Creates mucous and fluid lining of lungs, heart and throat
· Supports all forms of Kapha

Development

· Bhakti Yoga
· Moderate Diet
· Hatha Yoga

Disturbed

· Overweight
· Lung disorders
· Swollen glands
· Emotional attachment
· Excess phlegm

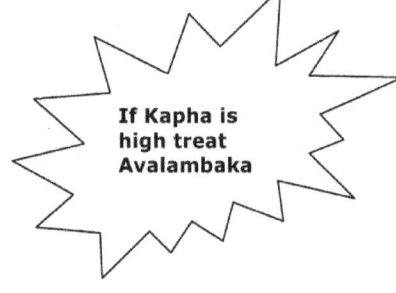

If Kapha is high treat Avalambaka

KEY SUBDOSHA IN TREATMENT

Tarpaka
Bodhaka
Kledaka
Sleshaka

S
U
P
P
O
R
T

Kledaka Kapha

Lubricates all digestion

balancing action of contents of g.i. tract

Principle Sites

· **STOMACH**

Governs

· Lubrication of the stomach and G.I. tract
· The alkaline secretions of the mucous membranes of stomach and G.I. tract

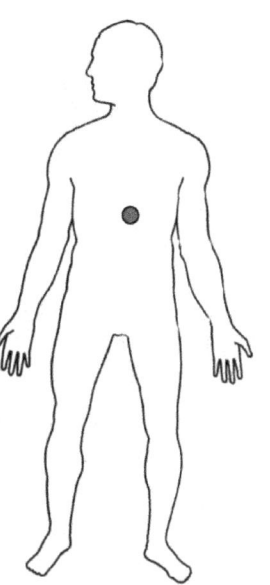

Gives

· Pleasure
· Stability to senses

Actions

· Lubricates the G.I. tract
· Balances Pitta and Vata in the G.I. tract
· Liquefies food

Development

· Fasting
· Moderate Diet
· Hatha Yoga

Disturbed

· Irregular secretion of stomach fluids
· Excess phlegm

Śleṣhaka Kapha

Lubricates all joints

outward going action (gives strength & stability)

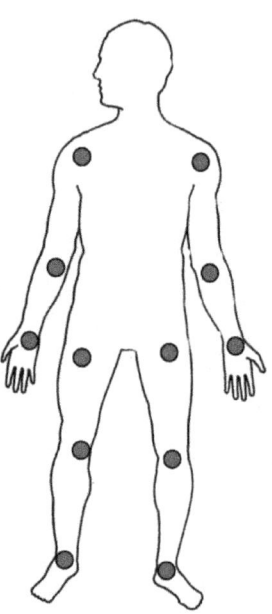

Principle Sites

· **JOINTS**

Governs

· Lubrication of the
synovial fluid
· Lubrication of tendons
and ligaments
· Movement due to
lubication

Gives

· Movment to the joints
· Stability to the body

Actions

· Holds joints together,
allowing for ease of
movement

Development

· Exercise
· Hatha Yoga

Disturbed

· Arthritic conditions
· Looseness of joints
· Too much causes
swelling of and
heaviness in the joints
· Too little of it causes
dry joints that are
difficult to move

Subtle forms of the Dosha—Prana, Tejas & Ojas

There is a concept in Ayurveda that the three dosha also have subtle or latent forms. The three manifest at the level of Ahamkara and the first diversification into an individual. Therefore, these subtle forms have a greater impact on the psychology than the three doshas which manifest at the Tanmatra level.

- Prana, Tejas and Ojas are the three vital essences that relate to the psychology
- They are the subtle forms, or positive essences of the doshas that function on the subtle (mental) and causal (Pranic) levels – above the Tanmatra level
- They are the positive essence of the doshas
- The doshas produce them when the doshas are healthy
- Ojas is transformed by Prana and Tejas in yoga practices, thus Ojas should be cultivated first.
- Ojas is the fuel, Tejas is the heat of Ojas, and Prana is the energy of Ojas.

Another opinion is that the subdosha of Vata, Prana Vayu, makes this form of Prana when healthy; the subdosha of Pitta, Sadhaka Pitta, makes the Tejas; and the subdosha of Kapha, Tarpaka Kapha, makes this kind of Ojas. As these subtle forms of the Tridosha are said to exist in the psychology (Manas) and manifest with the Ahamkara they are other divisions of the Maha Gunas; mainly relating to Sattva Guna.

Two Kinds of Ojas

The Caraka Samhita states that there are two kinds of Ojas:

1) One Ojas that lives in the heart and any reduction to it results in death, it is subtle and cannot be seen or known directly; it lives in the head and heart. Humans are born with 8 drops in the spiritual heart. These can be either strong or weak and this determines the overall vitality during the life of the person. These eight drops of Ojas are transmitted to the embryo during pregnancy and are fixed for life; if one drop is lost death results.

2) One Ojas that can be built up or depleted through meditation, food, lifestyle - this form relates directly to Kapha dosha and Dhatu metabolism. This form of Ojas is the one that can be increased through therapies. It is not fixed for life. It supports basic vitality and emotional stability. This Ojas helps use to resist disease and environmental changes. When speaking about Prana, Tejas and Ojas it is this type of Ojas that works with and supports Prana and Tejas.

Prana	Tejas	Ojas
Basic life-force of or vitality of the mind. Works through Prana Vayu on a gross level	Basic clarity of the mind, the light of our perceptions. Works through Sadhaka Pitta on a gross level	Basic mental stability and endurance in life. Works through Tarpaka Kapha on a gross level
Gives mental adaptability, capacity to communicate, coordination of thoughts, breadth of comprehension, enthusiasm, adaptability, creativity and strength, will to live, overall growth and evolution of body and mind.	Gives intelligence, reason, passion to learn or discover, zeal, power of self-discipline, capacity to perceive, courage, fearlessness, daring, boldness and valor.	Gives mental strength, contentment, patience, fortitude, calm, capacity for good memory and sustained concentration, peace of mind, strong immune system, physical endurance, capacity for sustained work and exertion.
Excess causes loss of mental control, sensory and motor coordination. Feel spaced out, ungrounded, like we are losing our sense of identity. Life-force loses its connection with the mind and body resulting in various incoherent behavior.	**Excess causes** overly critical and discriminating mind, delirium, negation of life experience, lack of satisfaction, overly pessimistic, excess doubt, anger, irritability, enmity.	**Excess causes** over contentment with life. Usually excess Ojas is not a problem. Excess prana and Tejas dry and burn up Ojas respectively. Excess prana and Tejas tend to manifest first and make low Ojas. Build Ojas if practicing Krya or Lala yoga.
Deficiency causes lack of mental energy, enthusiasm, curiosity, low life-force and healing energy, mind and senses become dull, heavy, without motivation.	**Deficiency causes** lack of capacity to inquire or discern, uncritical acceptance of things, difficult to digest experiences, overly passive, impressionable, easily influenced or dominated, lack in purpose or life-goal, fearful and low courage.	**Deficiency causes** lack of self-confidence and ability to concentrate, poor memory and lack in faith, no consistency to our thoughts or balance to our emotions. Nervous exhaustion or mental breakdowns may happen.

Deranging factors: drugs (medicinal or recreational), excess exposure to mass media influences or computers, too strong sensations, excess or pretend emotions, wrong meditation practices, excess breathing exercises can aggravate prana, psychedelic drugs can cause Tejas to burn too high. Generally wrong intake of impressions or wrong output of expressions derange the mind, which underlies or accompanies most diseases.

Balancing factors: meditation (esp. using breath, mantra together), prayer, self-study, deep sleep, deep relaxation. Being in nature and communion with the cosmic life-force in nature. Faith, love, receptivity, compassion and understanding are also important to develop.

Chapter Five Study Questions

1. What are the differences between the sub-dosha and the primary dosha?

2. What does Vata dosha not control?

3. Why does Vata control sweating?

4. Which sub-dosha of Vata brings the nutrients to the digestion?

5. Which of the follow polarities of Vata's sub-doshas is wrong?

6. Sadhaka Pitta is responsible for what processes of the body?

7. Which form of Pitta controls the main digestive metabolism?

8. Which form of Kapha controls the primary function of lubrication?

9. Sleshaka Kapha is responsible for what function?

10. What are Prana, Tejas and Ojas?

CHAPTER SIX
THE SEVEN DHATU

The three Doshas, are the primary foundations of Ayurveda because they categorize *functions* into three classifications. The "five states of matter" which they control are representing the structural aspect of the body. Thus, the five groups of matter which mold structure are not actually "things" as much as they are groups of matter that have similar "functions". Nature has a law that: "form follows function". This can be seen in nature in many ways, for example how the movement of wind modifies the form and structure of trees, sand, rocks, etc. Hence, Dhatu follow Dosha as Dosha are the function and Dhatu are the form or structure.

Here is the classic definition of Anatomy and Physiology in Ayurveda:

dosa-dhātu-malā mūlam sadā dehasya tam calah |

"Doshas, Dhatus and Malas are the foundation of the body throughout life."
AS.SU.11.1

After the three Doshas there are four primary divisions in Ayurvedic anatomy – Dhatus (tissues), Srotas (channels), Malas (waste products) and Kalas (membranes that define and separate). Animating these functions and physical structures are Prana, Agni and Ojas. In Ayurvedic texts the Dhatus include the organs, glands, channels (Srota) and membranes (Kala).

Dosha	functions in the body that allow elements in and out of the body
Dhatu	the structural aspect of the body built by nutrients
Mala	the waste products produced by correct metabolism (function)

In the practical application there is a difference in diagnosis and treatment between Dhatu and Srota. Therefore, in this course we will study both independently. The Kalas can be seen as a part of Dhatu and the diagnosis and treatment of a Dhatu will correct any problem of the Kala. However, the Kala have an important role and there will be a lesson on them as well in this course. Prana, Agni and Ojas represent the vital intelligence of the body (prana); the capacity to transform matter (Agni); and the ultimate nourishment received from nature (Ojas). Each of these three has a general function in the body and a specific function in the Dhatus.

Following Dosha the most important element in Ayurvedic anatomy is the concept of Dhatu. The Sanskrit word *Dhatu* means "root" or "support". It comes from the root word *DU* in Sanskrit. The current definition of Dhatu is: *"That which supports (Dharana) and which nourishes (Poshana)".*

"That which nourishes the next Dhatu and supports the body is known as Dhatu. That means that the Upadhatu (sub-tissue) can support, but not nourish, therefore, Upadhatu cannot nourish any level of the body"

The above definition implies that the Dhatus are the primary factors in both physiology and nourishment. It also points out that the Upadhatu, or the sub tissue, that is produced by the Dhatu cannot be considered a Dhatu by itself as it cannot nourish other Dhatus. Additionally, Dosha cannot be called Dhatu as they cannot fulfill the two requirements of support and nourishment. By the same definition Mala also cannot be Dhatu as it can neither support or nourish the body. Hence, only the seven Dhatu can be called "*Dhatu*" by the above definition.

The Dhatus become the sites of disease as they are the structural - as opposed the functional - aspect of anatomy. In a normal state they support the physical structure and form of the body. In a diseased state they fail to support both the physical structure and as a result health.

According to Ayurveda there are seven Dhatu. These seven levels of tissue development are *not like an onion* that represent layers of the body. They are actually indicating seven levels of structural development from nutrients consumed by the body. In other words, the Dhatu are a direct result of our nutritional and respiratory intake. Whatever is taken into the body through the lungs or digestion will either support or destroy Dhatu development. The Dhatus demonstrate an increasing complex metabolism of nutrients. These nutrients become more and more refined as they go on to develop the next Dhatu. This is the primary concept of the Dhatu.

The Dhatu are always listed in the follow order because this is the order of nutrient metabolism:

1) Rasadhātu   (Plasma -including blood plasma- and Lymphatic tissues)
2) Raktadhātu   (Red Blood cells / Heat in general)
3) Māmsadhātu   (Muscle tissue)
4) Medadhātu   (Fat and adipose tissue)
5) Asthidhātu   (Bone tissue)
6) Majjādhātu   (Bone Marrow and Nerve tissue)
7) Shukradhātu   (Reproductive tissue)

According to this idea Rasa Dhatu is the foundation of the body and the other six Dhatus. The Dhatu concept has less to do with one tissue actually "building the next" tissue, but more precisely that our nutritional intake is progressively refined through each level of tissue metabolism.

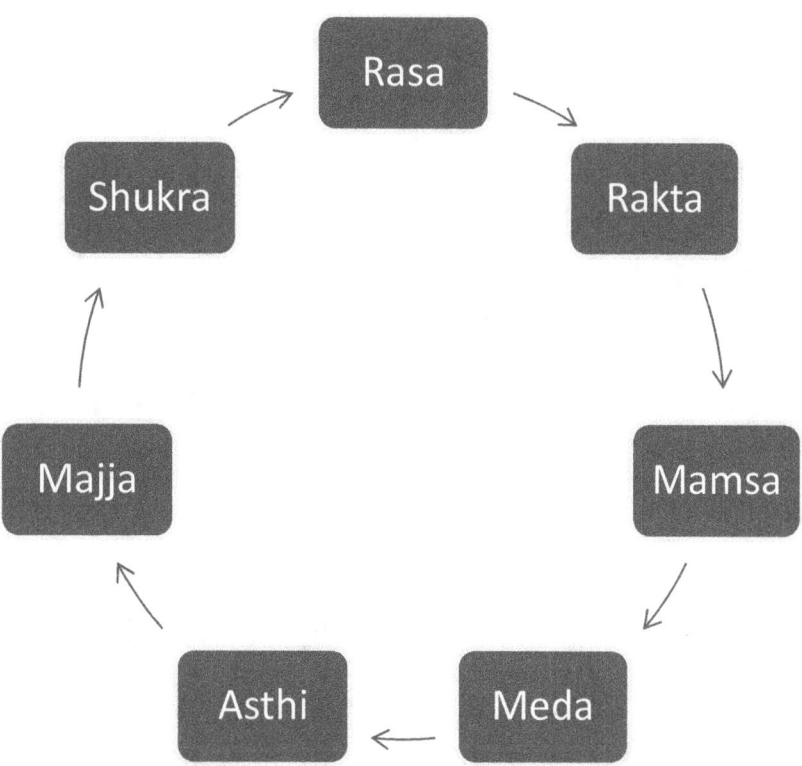

This means that if one tissue becomes malnourished through poor diet the succeeding tissues will also suffer some form of malnutrition over time. Obviously diet plays a central role in the health of the tissues as they are built directly from food, which means the five elements. On the other hand if the nutritional intake is good then the tissues will be in a stronger state to resist disease if a disorder should try to lodge itself in a Dhatu. We use the word "tissues" here to represent those physical places of the body, not necessarily muscle or skin that we would normally associate with the word "tissue". We consider blood, for example, a "tissue" because it is formed from our consumption of food, not because it is in a layer or a certain place of the body.

Once again the idea of 'structure and form' has to be placed aside when trying to understand the logic of Ayurvedic anatomy as related to the Dhatu formation. Each tissue builds not only itself but also the succeeding tissue. This begins with the first tissue, Rasadhatu or plasma, and then continues through all seven Dhatus. The seventh Dhatu forms Ojas which then nourishes all the other Dhatus forming a dynamic cycle. The main source of nutrition for the first tissue is food and water.

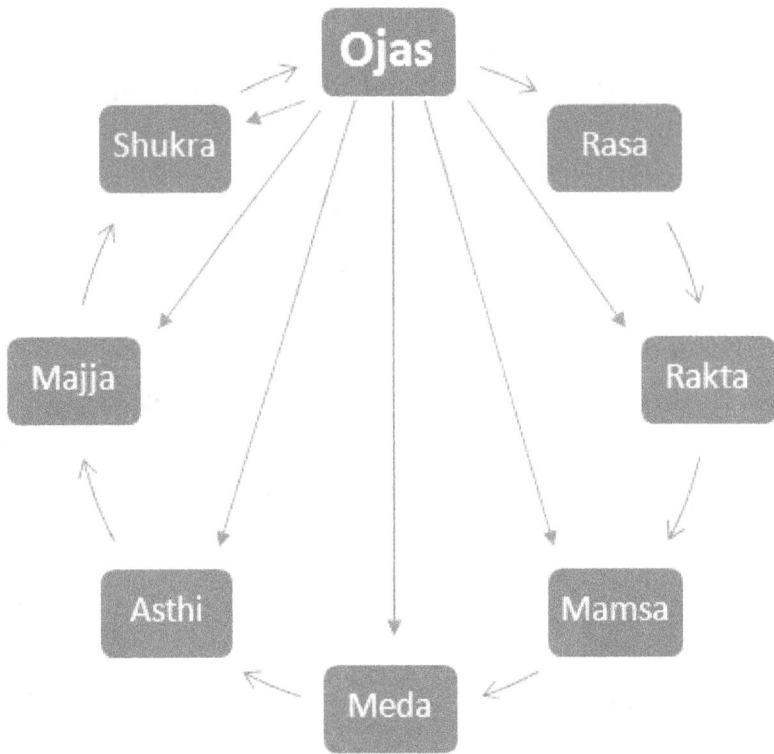

In each level the food and drink consumed by the body becomes more refined and nourishes each subsequent level in its turn. Each Dhatu becomes more atomic or potent. The ultimate potency in the human body is the ability to create life. Thus, the reproductive fluids (ovum and sperm) are considered to be the highest, most refined, product of the body. They make up the seventh level of the body or Shukradhatu.

The last Dhatu also produces a substance known in Ayurveda as Ojas. Ojas is the primal energy of the body and goes back through the cycle of the seven tissues to nourish all of the levels of the body (see the diagram above). Many modern Ayurvedic doctors that are trained in both Allopathy (modern medicine) and Ayurveda state that Ojas is our basic immunity. In other words, when Ojas is low our immune system is low. The concept of Ojas is also directly related to fertility. According to Ayurveda a strong, health seventh level and Ojas must exist in order for conception to produce a strong healthy child.

Not only does each level nourish the next level and its sub-levels, it also has a specific waste product. The secondary tissues and waste products are important because they can give us an indication of our health. For example, they manifest as hair, nails and body odor. A healthy Dhatu produces a healthy "waste". For example: if you have excessive discharges in the eyes then it indicates imbalances in Majjadhatu.

Each Dhatu has one or more sub-tissues (Upadhatu) as well a waste product (Mala) that is produced from the Dhatu metabolism. See the table below:

Dhatu	Upadhatu	Dhatu Mala
Rasa plasma and lymph fluids	-top layer of skin -menstrual flow -breast milk	-poshaka Kapha -mucus
Rakta red blood cells	-blood vessels -small tendons	-poshaka Pitta -bile
Mamsa muscles	-six layers of skin -small ligaments	-accumulation in body cavities, i.e., navel, ear wax, smegma, etc.
Meda fat and adipose tissues	-large tendons -large ligaments	-sweat
Asthi bones	-teeth	-nails -hair
Majja Bone marrow and nerves	-tears	-sclerotic fluid in the eyes
Shukra reproductive fluids	-none	-none (or pubic hair)
Ojas primary energy	-none	none

Some Ayurvedic people state that Ojas is the upadhatu of Shukra. This is a problem if we follow the definition that was given above - and which is taught in the Ayurvedic universities in India - because Ojas is both a support and nourishes all Dhatus. By this definition it cannot be an upadhatu. Thus, Ojas is a separate substance that is neither Dosha, Dhatu or Mala.

Each Dhatu has two components, one stable (sthayi) and the other in ongoing development or unstable (asthayi). These two aspects of Dhatu nutrition and metabolism form the foundation of Ayurvedic physiology.

The formative or instable part (asthayi) of the tissue turns into the stable form (sthayi) by the action of the Dhatu Agni located in the Kala (membrane). The stable part (sthayi) stays in the dhatu and helps to form and maintain the tissue. This is the metabolic process that converts the asthayi to sthayi. From this process of metabolism secondary tissues (Upadhatus) and waste materials (Malas) are produced. The end result of this metabolic process is the formation of a new asthayi that goes on to nourish the next Dhatu.

For example, after the formative Rasa (asthayi rasa), produces the stable Rasa and its secondary tissue (Upadhatu), as well as its waste material (Mala), there is a subtler form of Rasa left over which becomes the formative tissue for Rakta (asthayi Rakta), the next Dhatu in the body. Thus, we see an ongoing cycle of nourishment in the seven Dhatus that results in the creation of Ojas.

There are several components to correct Dhatu function or physiology:
1. dhatu structure with its own attributes
2. nutrients coming into the dhatu (Asthayi)
3. metabolism of the nutrients (Agni)
4. result of metabolism (Upadhatu, Mala & Sthayi)
5. the dhatu is maintained by the correct metabolism (Sthayi)
6. this metabolism creates a refined nutrient for the next dhatu (Asthayi)

By this same logic the impairment of nutrition to one Dhatu will be reflected in the next Dhatu. It takes time but eventually all proceeding Dhatus can become effected when one preceding Dhatu is not metabolizing correctly. The correct formation of any tissue depends upon two factors; the previous tissue must be properly metabolized and the Agni of the tissue must be normal and balanced.

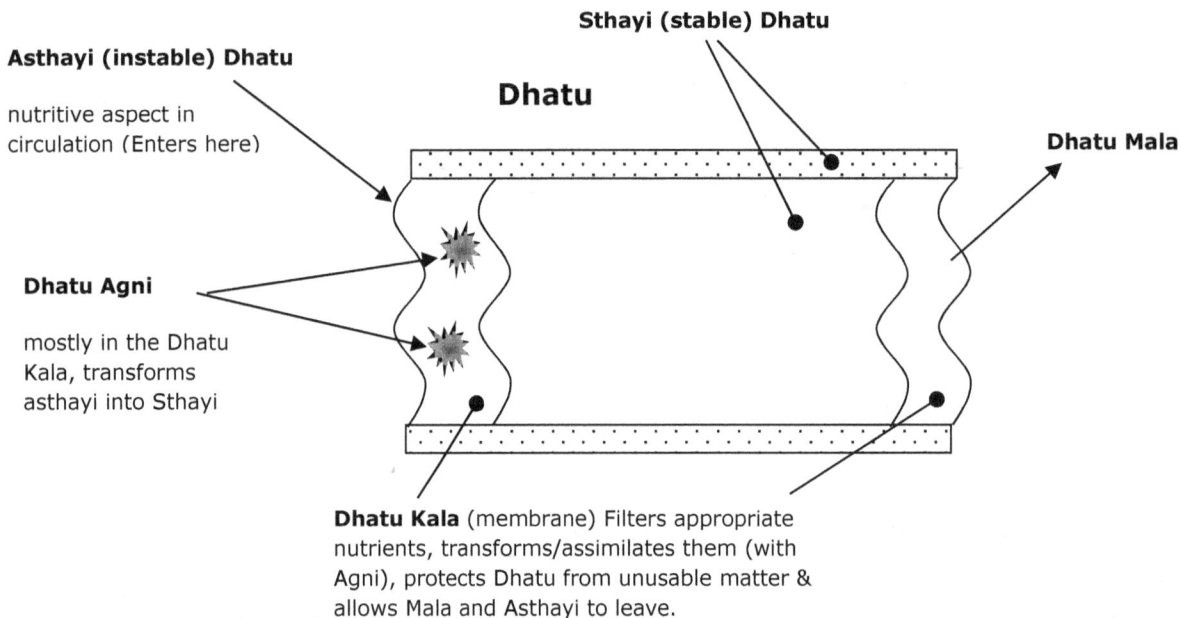

If the tissue Agni (dhatu Agni) is too low too much of the tissue will be produced and its quality will be low. If the tissue Agni is too high, too little of the tissue will be produced. Proper metabolism is achieved when the following three things are correct:

1. Agni is balanced
2. Nutrients are correct
3. Waste products are removed

It is the three Doshas that perform the above three functions to allow Dhatu metabolism to function correctly. If the Dosha are not working correctly then the Dhatus will not be formed correctly.

Dhatu Metabolism - Dhātu parināma

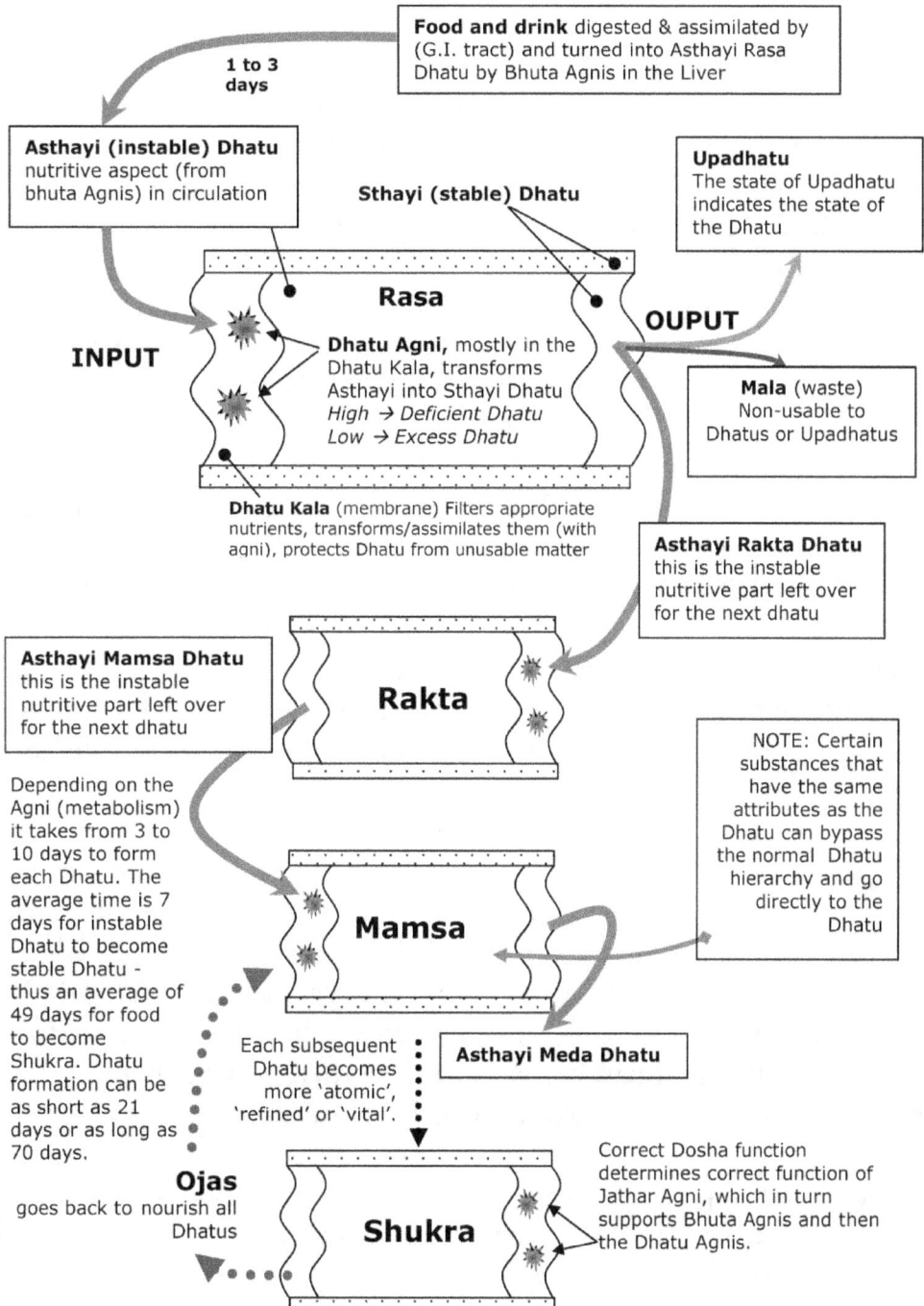

Description of the Seven Dhatus

Rasadhātu

The function of Rasadhatu is to give satisfaction (trupi), luster (prasannata) and nourishment (prana) to the body. Rasa provides nutrition to all the tissues. It is responsible for hydration and maintaining the pH balance of the tissues. Rasa is responsible for the formation of Raktadhatu.

The Mula Sthana of Rasa is the Hridayam (heart) and has 24 Srotas that carry or hold Rasa. Ten to the upper body, ten to the lower body and four to the trunk or central area of the body. Rasadhatu pervades the entire body through the plasma, blood, lymphatic system, skin and mucous membranes. Rasadhatu is controlled and formed mainly by Kapha.

The dominate Gunas of Rasa are: Drava (liquid), Sara (flowing), Manda (slow), Snigdha (unctuous), Picchilla (slimy).

Rasa can be defined as: the or juice of plants, of fruit any liquid or fluid, the best or finest or prime part of anything, essence, water, liquor, drink, juice of the sugar-cane, syrup, any mixture, draught, elixir, potion, melted, nectar, a constituent fluid or essential juice of the body, serum, the primary juice called *chyle* (formed from the food and changed by the bile into blood), mercury, quicksilver (sometimes regarded as a kind of quintessence of the human body, elsewhere as the seminal fluid of Shiva, semen virile, any mineral or metallic salt, a metal or mineral in a state of fusion, taste, flavor as the principal quality of fluids.

By the above definition of the word Rasa it is apparent that it is a primary substance that supports and nourishes the body / mind organism. It represents the essence of the human being and through it all physical structure is maintained.

When Rasa is sufficient we feel happiness and contentment. We have a sense of fullness in life and vitality and enjoy participating in life. Rasa gives a love for life and a sense of beauty and happiness.

Note that the terms "plasma" or "lymph" is often used for Rasadhatu. Be aware that Rasa also means the plasma found in the blood. So Rasadhatu is not limited to the lymphatic system as it also includes the blood plasma. This is a source of confusion for many people. This concept is very important because it explains how the nutrients digested in the liver get to Rasadhatu first, before Raktadhatu. If we think of Rasadhatu as lymph or plasma limited to the non-blood liquid portions of the body this nutrient transfer would be impossible. It is through the "blood" that Rasadhatu carries all the nutrients throughout the body. Hence, the words "lymph", "plasma" and "blood" can be confusing when trying to understand Rasadhatu.

Rasadhatu can be built up by liquids and foods that are slightly oily. Other things that build Rasa are sour fruit juices, dairy products, particularly Ghee and milk. Basically, all food that is wholesome will nourish Rasa.

> **Dhatu**: RASA (Plasma)
> **Upadhatu**: Tvak (skin) 1st layer, Ārtava (menstruation), Stanya (lactation)
> **Mala**: Kapha
>
> - Rasa means 'essence, 'juice', 'nectar'
> - Rasa supports the whole body with nutritious fluid
> - Main organ of rasa is the first layer of skin, which is the main organ of the body thus we can read the state of rasa from the skin
> - Rasa is easily modified by the diet
> - Linked to immune function along with Rakta and Majja.

Raktadhātu

The main function of Raktadhatu is to support the human body. It is responsible for promotion of strength, complexion, happiness, nutrition to the next dhatu (Mamsa) and a long life to the body. Rakta plays a vital role is transporting nutrients, prana and heat throughout the body. Rakta also maintains the *Ten Vital Organs* of Ayurveda: the two temples, heart, head, bladder, throat, blood, reproductive fluid, Ojas and rectum. These Ten Vital Organs are a concept in Ayurveda relating to the most fragile areas of the body – if these areas are damaged then life leaves the body. Hence, they are protected and given special attention in treatments.

The Mula Sthana of Rakta is the liver and spleen. It lives in all the blood vessels and so permeates the whole body through veins and arteries. It fills the Dhatus and gives them nutrition.

The dominate Gunas of Rakta are: Drava (liquid), Sara (flowing), Manda (slow), Snigdha (unctuous), Mrudhu (soft), Picchchila (slimy), Madhura (sweet), Lavanam (salty).

> **Dhatu**: RAKTA (Blood)
> **Upadhatu**: Śirā (blood vessels), Kandara (small tendons and sinews)
> **Mala**: Pitta
>
> - Rakta supports the body through providing nutrients
> - Rakta = Hemoglobin which is responsible for the transportation of oxygen thus provides energy to the body
> - Rakta circulates heat to the entire body
> - Linked to immune function along with rasa and Majja

When our blood is sufficient the body has abundant energy. Rakta gives happiness, intelligence, peace, tolerance for stress and tenderness (emotionally). *Rakta* literally means what is colored or what is red – this means that Rakta is the Hemoglobin in the blood and not the "blood" in a general sense. The Rakta gives us color and heat to the body. It is transformed from Rasa by Samana Vayu and by Ranjaka Pitta. It contains Pitta dosha and

Pitta is responsible to build and maintain Raktadhatu.

Raktadhatu can be built up by dark green leafy vegetables, whole grains, carrots, beets, and by red meat.

Mamsadhatu

The function of Mamsadhatu is to give strength and nourishment. It is responsible for nourishing Medadhatu. Mamsa has a binding (lepana) effect on the body structure and holds it together. The muscles serve to cover and give strength to our basic bodily frame. Mamsa protect the body from injury and harm by its covering. Mamsadhatu gives the body the capacity for work, movement and action.

The Mula Sthana of Mamsa is the joints of the body where there are veins and arteries. Mamsa appears in many forms (large, small, thick, thin, flat round, etc.) depending on the need and location. Mamsa is adapted to different needs with the help of Vata Dosha.

The dominate Gunas of Mamsa are: Stula (gross), Sthira (static), Guru (heavy), Khara (rough), Kathina (hard), Shlakshna (smooth).

When Mamsa is sufficient we have courage, confidence and strength, along with the capacity for openness, forgiveness and happiness. The term "mamsa" itself comes from the root "mam" meaning to hold firm.

Mamsadhatu can be built up by whole grains, by foods with high earth and water content (roots, beans, nuts, etc.), dairy products and by meat.

Dhatu: MAMSA (Muscles)
Upadhatu: Small Ligaments, Tvak (Skin, 6 sub-layers)
Mala: wastes that accumulate in orifices

- Gives support and protection to the body
- Binds and holds the body together
- Skin (6 sub-layers) relates to Mamsa Upadhatu.
- Adapts to the function or need of the body depending on location

---

Medadhātu

The function of Meda is to provide lubrication (snehana), perspiration (sveda), strength (drudhatva) and nourishment (pusti) to Asthidhātu. Meda provides insulation to the body and protects it from heat and cold. Meda dhatu provides nutrients and energy for emergency situations. It provides a layer of protection from shock or accidents and offers and additional protection to the vital organs in the trunk are of the body.

The Mula Sthana of Meda is the abdomen. Meda pervades the body but is concentrated in the lower back, thighs, breasts and buttocks. It provides lubrication to all tissues.

The dominate Gunas of Meda are: Drava (liquid), Sulakshna (smooth).

Meda helps lubricate the throat and give a melodious voice. Meda gives a good skin, hair and complexion. Fat gives a sense of contentment, smoothness and happiness. Some people can become obese to counter a feeling of not being loved, as Meda provides the sense of contentment and love. The word "Medas" means what is oily.

Medadhatu can be built up by vegetable fats like sesame oil or by animal fats like butter, ghee, cheese, lard, fish (oily) and meat.

Dhatu: MEDA (Fat)
Upadhatu: Snāyu (large tendons, large ligaments)
Mala: Sveda (Sweat)

- Meda provides lubrication and protection
- Gives strength and energy in emergencies
- Insulates body from hot and cold

Asthidhātu

The function of Asthi is support (dharana). The bones serve to uphold all our tissues and give them firmness and a strong foundation. They are the strongest Dhatu in the body and are the last to be destroyed. They support all tendons and ligaments in the body.

The Mula Sthana of Asthi is the colon. Asthi is of five types in Ayurveda. They are five groups of Asthi which are as follows - flat and wide (kapalasthi), teeth (ruchakashti), cartilage (tarunasthi), short and irregular bones (valayasthi), and long bones (nalakasthi). Ayurveda considers that they are 360 bones in the body, Sushruta eliminates some types and give the total as 300.

The dominate Gunas of Asthi are: Guru (heavy), Khara (rough), Kathina (hard), Sthula (gross), Sthira (static).

When Asthi is sufficient we have stability, confidence, security and stamina. The spaces or porous areas in the bone hold Vata Dosha. Vata is responsible to build and maintain Asthidhatu. The word "Asthi" comes from the root "stha", which means to stand or endure.

Asthidhatu can be built up by whole grains, dark leafy green vegetables, seaweed, and any food that nourishes Meda Dhatu.

Dhatu: ASHTI (Bone)
Upadhatu: Danta (teeth)
Mala: Nakha (nails), Keśa (hair on head), Loma (body hair).

- Provides support for body
- Strongest dhatu in the body
- Hollow part of bone is filled with Vatadosha

Majjādhātu

The function of Majjadhatu is to give contentment (purana), satisfaction or pleasure to the body and mind. Majja provides oily or unctuous qualities to the bone (Asthi) and to the body in general. It provides strength. As bone marrow Majja serves to fill the empty spaces in bone. Majja as nerve and brain tissue fills the spaces and provides a tissue pathway for electric impulses of Vata Dosha. Majja also provides for the production of synovial fluid that reduces friction between the articular cartilage of synovial joints during movement. It aids in the lubrication of the eyes, nerves and brain.

The Mula Sthana of Majja is the thigh bones. Majja existing in all bones as the bone marrow and throughout the body as nerve tissue. Majja is the tissue structure of the nervous system - NOT the movement of nerve impulse in the tissue. Majja is of two kinds; red and white. The Red Majja has Pitta in it and produces red blood cells; it resides mainly in smaller, spongy bones. Part of these red blood cells are transformed into white blood cells. The Yellow Majja lives more in the long, larger bones.

The dominate Gunas of Majja are: Snigdha (unctuous), Mridu (soft).

Majja gives us a sense of fullness and completion in life. When it is deficient it creates a feeling of emptiness and anxiety. Majja provides the body and mind with affection, love and compassion by its lubricating nature. "Majja" comes from the root "maj", to sink, as the nerve tissue is sunk deep in the bones.

Majja can be built up by ghee, butter, seeds, nuts, vegetable oils, animal fat and marrow. Meat and fish have some effect on Majja as well.

Dhatu: MAJJA (Bone marrow, nerve)
Upadhatu: Asru (secretion from eyes)
Mala: Netra Sneha (unctuousness of eyes)

- Majja gives give contentment and satisfaction to mind & body
- Majja "fills" the bones and stabilizes Vatadosha
- Endocrine system function that is metabolic in nature is linked to Majja
- Majja creates red blood cells, some of which are transformed into white blood cells that are linked to immune function

---

Shukradhātu

The function of Shukra is reproduction (garbha utpadana). Shukra allows us to produce life. There are eight factors that allow the manifestation of Shukra - excitement, passionate desire, fluidity, sliminess, heaviness, anubhava (atomic properties), the tendency to move outward and the movement of Apana vayu. Shukra only manifests its full capacity during puberty. Prior to puberty Shukra is present everywhere in the body but is not yet manifest; Caraka says that like a flower that blooms long after the plant has been alive; so too, Shukra is the flower of the human physical development.

The Mula Sthana of Shukra is Majjadhatu. Shukra exists everywhere in the body and allows us to feel the sensation of touch. If there is a lack of sensation someplace then Shukra is deficient in that place.

The dominate Gunas of Shukra are: Drava (liquid), Snigdha (unctuous), Guru (heavy), Madhura (sweet).

Shukra means the sperm and ovum, and means reproductive fluids in general. Shukra specifically indicates the male sperm and Artava is used to indicate the female ovum. In most texts the two are grouped together under the term *shukra.*

Shukra provides patience, strength, energy and stamina for the entire body. It supports the immune system and all other Dhatus. It gives light to the eyes and inspiration. Shukra produces Ojas when it is healthy and abundant. The word "Shukra" itself means "seed" and "luminous".

Shukradhatu can be built up by Ghee, milk, raw sugar, seeds, nuts, vegetable oils, eggs and animal fats.

Dhatu: SHUKRA (Reproductive, Fertility) **Upadhatu**: none **Mala**: none
• Shukra provides support to all other dhatus • Shukra provides patience, strength and stamina • Shukra allows reproduction and pleasure • Endocrine system function related to growth is linked to Shukra • Shukra allows the sense of touch in the body

The Three Doshas as Mala of the Dhatus

It is important to understand that Rasa and Rakta dhatus produce a preliminary form of Kapha and Pitta called *Poshaka* Kapha and *Poshaka* Pitta. These are nutrient states or preliminary states of Kapha Dosha and Pitta Dosha. The *poshaka* Mala are responsible for the increase or decrease of both Kapha and Pitta as they form a nutrient like the Dosha. Once the Prana, or intelligence, of the Dosha mixes with the poshaka Mala it becomes part of the Dosha.

This means that Kapha and Pitta produce Rasa and Rakta and are also their waste materials. In normal amounts they help produce these tissues. In excess they appear as a significant amount of Mala and excess Dosha. When these two Dhatus are overdeveloped these two Dosha will be produced in excess. This has a tendency to involve Kapha in most diseases of Rasa and Pitta in most diseases of Rakta.

Vata Dosha is not a waste material of the bone. Vata is generally produced as various gases in the body. One sutra in Caraka states that the Mala of Asthi (left over from the metabolism of Asthi controlled by Vata) is an upward moving gas that lodges in the small intestine or stomach. In other words, this Vata Mala is responsible for indigestion.

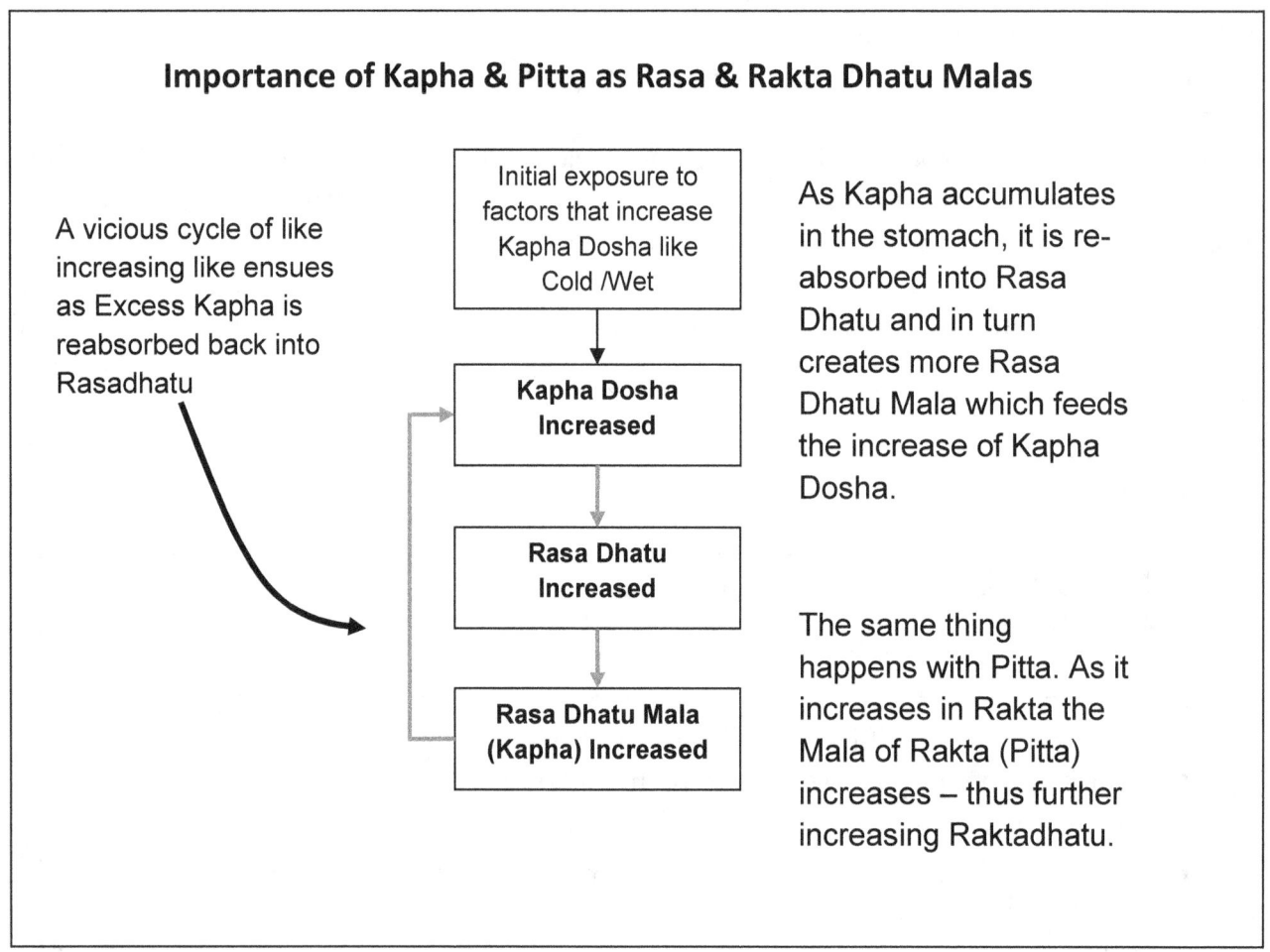

Importance of Kapha & Pitta as Rasa & Rakta Dhatu Malas

A vicious cycle of like increasing like ensues as Excess Kapha is reabsorbed back into Rasadhatu

Initial exposure to factors that increase Kapha Dosha like Cold /Wet

Kapha Dosha Increased

Rasa Dhatu Increased

Rasa Dhatu Mala (Kapha) Increased

As Kapha accumulates in the stomach, it is re-absorbed into Rasa Dhatu and in turn creates more Rasa Dhatu Mala which feeds the increase of Kapha Dosha.

The same thing happens with Pitta. As it increases in Rakta the Mala of Rakta (Pitta) increases – thus further increasing Raktadhatu.

Look at this cycle represented in the diagram above.

The following points are important to fully understand Dosha, Dhatu, Mala.
- Dhatus are the result of food being digestion & assimilated.
- Food we eat either become Ama (toxins) or nutritive pre-tissue substance.
- This nutritive pre-tissue substance is called instable (asthayi) and forms the first dhatu – Rasa.
- Correct nourishment and a good Agni (digestion) create a high quality dhatu.
- Doshas control the formation of dhatus.
- Doshas are cause of disease, dhatus are **the location of disease**. However, if dhatu is healthy and strong, it is impossible for disease to get a foothold.
- Mind affects dhatu health through the doshas.

For your reference here is a diagram of the seven layers of skin in Ayurveda and a correlation to modern anatomy. The Seven level are called:

1. Avabhasini
2. Lohita
3. Sveta
4. Tamara
5. Vedhini
6. Rohini
7. Mamsadhara

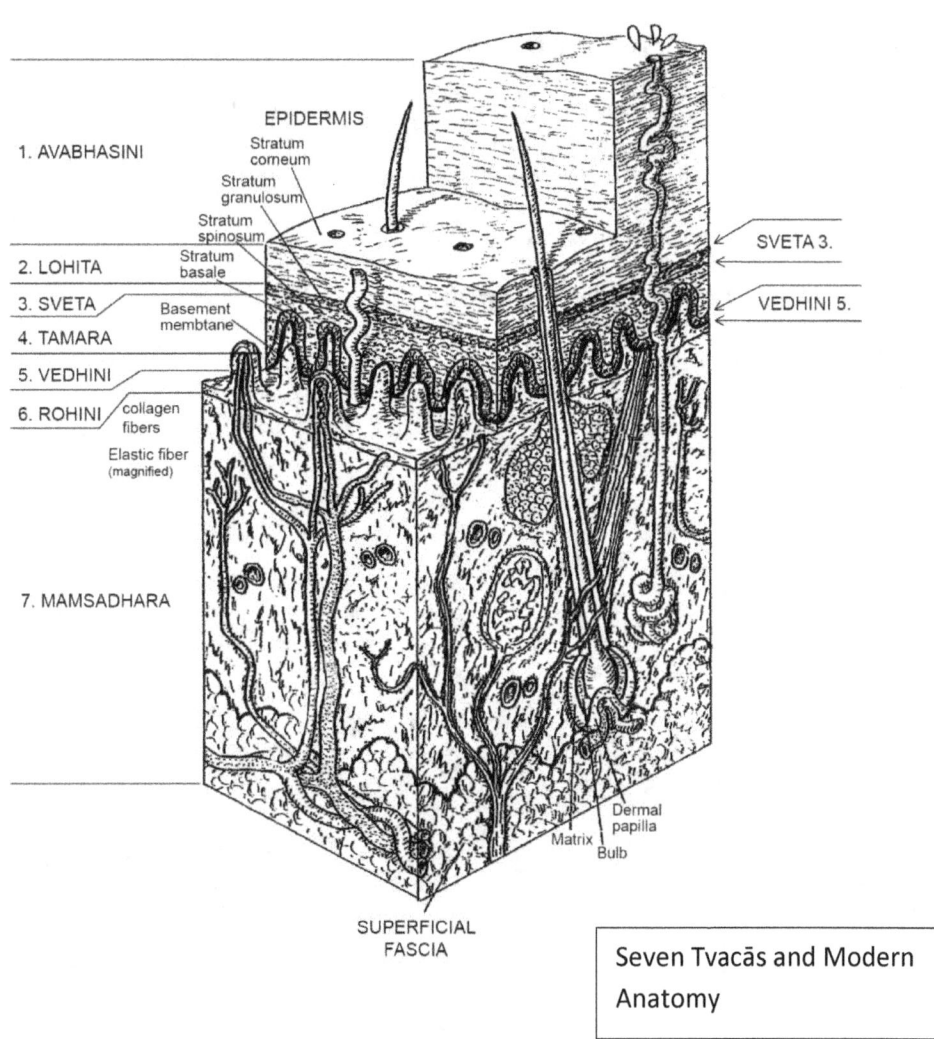

TVACAS

Seven Tvacās and Modern Anatomy

Study Questions for Chapter Six

1. What are the foundations of the body throughout life?

2. What is the definition of Dhatu?

3. The Dhatus demonstrate an increasing refined metabolism of nutrients; what does this result in?

4. The formative part (asthayi) of the tissue turns into the stable form (sthayi). What happens to the stable part (sthayi)?

5. What is the primary function of Rasa Dhatu?

6. Why is Rakta dhatu's main function to be "support of the human body"?

7. What is the primary function of Meda dhatu?

8. Majja dhatu has two aspects; what are they?

9. Shukra manifests at what time during the development of the body?

10. What does Ojas, the primal energy of the body, come from?

CHAPTER SEVEN
AGNI, AMA & MALA

Besides the three Dosha and seven Dhatu, there are two important Ayurvedic principles that we must consider: *Agni* and *Āma*. People wrongly assume that whatever they put into their mouths will be used by the body in some beneficial way. This is not true. The digestion and assimilation of nutrients depends on enzyme function. In Ayurveda the concept of enzyme function is the most important factor in nutrition. The Sanskrit work for this enzyme function is *Agni* – which literally means 'fire' or something that *'transforms one thing into another'*.

What are enzymes? They are special proteins in the body that bind themselves to other particles for the purpose of transforming them into something else. Enzymes speed up biological processes in the body. Most of them have very specific actions and roles in the body. They help to transform nutrients in the body without being altered or used up in the process. They are concerned in all digestive and cellular processes. However, they are quite sensitive and can be disabled by excess acidity or alkaline (pH) in the body. Hence, if your digestion is too acidic or too alkaline the enzyme function will be retarded or even stopped.

Enzymes are a field of major study in the biochemical world. Many medicines are made that either inhibit or accelerate different enzyme productions in the body. The role of enzymes was almost ignored for many years in modern science and nutrition, but their possible use to target medicines to specific locations in the body has opened up the coffers of the research industry. The digestive enzymes hold the key not only to proper nutrient assimilation, but your health in general.

In the body the Agni is controlled by the three Doshas. Agni is directly controlled by Pachaka Pitta, Samana Vata and Kledaka Kapha in that order. As Pitta is also called 'fire' it is important to ask: "What is the difference between Agni and Pitta Dosha?" *Agni is used by Pitta* because Pitta is an intelligent manager that controls two states of matter: fire and water. Agni is therefore the 'fire' aspect of Pitta Dosha. Agni cannot 'use' Pitta because Pitta is the intelligence that gives more or less 'fire' to Agni when it is needed. Pitta is helped in this work to control Agni by Vata and Kapha who provide wind and protective mucus to control this form of pure fire. Hence, one thing to remember is that the Doshas modify the Agnis. Agni does not modify Dosha!

The concept of Agni (enzymes) in Ayurveda is well defined. There are thirteen different groups of Agni; the primary Agni in the duodenum, the five elemental Agni in the liver, and seven cellular Agni that work in the seven Dhatus; (1+5+7=13).

Primary Agni (Jathara Agni) – literally *"digestive fire in the stomach"*.

There is ONE of these agnis which is a group of several different enzymes. It relates to the enzymes that are mainly collected in the duodenum, but also include enzymes in the lower stomach. This agni controls all enzymes from the lower stomach to the rectum, though usually it is said that Jathara agni 'lives in the duodenum'. These enzymes (agnis) are secreted by the stomach, liver, gall bladder, pancreas and small intestine membrane. They begin to transform food sent down from the stomach. Jathara Agni is responsible for the transformation of food into macro nutrients (proteins, carbohydrates and fats) that are then absorbed into the bloodstream and taken directly to the liver and the next set of agnis. This agni also helps in the micro nutrient absorption that takes place in the large intestine or colon. Jathara Agni also acts as our first level of defence against ingested pathogens such as bacteria, viruses or parasites.

Elemental Agnis (Pañca Bhūta Agni) – literally *"the five element fires"*.

There are FIVE groups of these agnis, one for each of the five Bhuta or elements. This is the enzyme function in the liver. Once food has undergone the first phase of digestion in the small intestines, the nutritive aspect of food (called *Ahara Rasa* or chyle in modern terms) gets absorbed through the mucus membrane into the blood stream and carried to the liver. The liver then transforms this nutritive into the first Dhatu, Rasadhatu. It is here that these five groups of Bhuta agnis fully transform the macro and micro nutrients received from the G.I. tract. This is the 'second stage of transformation'.

Cellular Agnis (Dhātva Agni) – literally *"the tissue digestive fires"*.

There are SEVEN groups of these agnis, one for each Dhatu. This is the final level of Agni function that corresponds to the enzyme function at a cellular level in the Dhatu. These agnis are responsible for basic cellular metabolism. The Dhatus have different kinds of agnis depending on the type of Dhatu. For example, Rakta Dhatu Agni will need to be different than Asthi Dhatu Agni because the tissues are different and have different needs.

These three groups of thirteen agnis form a hierarchy whereby each subsequent level depends on the correct functioning of the previous level. This means that the Agni in the digestive tract, Jathara Agni, supports the Pancha Bhuta Agnis and the Dhatu Agnis (Dhātva Agni). This means that if you want to modify the Dhatu Agnis all you need to do is change the main Agni in the G.I. tract and the liver and Dhatu Agnis will have to follow the main agni.

The importance of the primary Agni function in the small intestine cannot be overstated. If either the duodenum or liver Agni (enzymes) are affected then it causes a ripple effect that suppresses the ability to digest most kinds of foods. Ayurveda states that if this enzyme function is strong then the person will have good health because they will be able to assimilate what foods they do consume – even if they are of poor quality. So according to this insight a strong Agni is more important than the food quality – although poor food will eventually weaken Agni.

Digestion is the process that acts on everything ingested into the mouth and transforms it to become part of the body. Everything that comes in to the body, food, bacteria, pollutants, etc., has to be treated by the digestive process. Hence, the extraction of nutritive parts (macro and micro nutrients) and the elimination of the unwanted parts (pathogens, insoluble fibre, waste, etc.) is collectively called the "digestion". This process has several aspects; *identification, separation, assimilation and evacuation.* All these things are the are the domain of Agni. The three Doshas control Agni and allow Agni to function correctly.

Agni is not only about digesting food, it also provides a protective role which contributes to our overall immunity. This is part of the intelligent function of Agni which we call "identification". It is able to identify nutritive food, non-nutritive food, pathogens, toxins and waste materials. This is a very specific role of Agni and should never be forgotten. Thanks to Agni we do not ingest poison substances. Agni can also 'burn up' pathogens and other toxins when needed. If it is not able to do this it rejects the food by vomiting, or in some cases by diarrhea. Thus, Agni is our 'first' immunity in many respects.

Assessing the state of the Agni function in the body is very important in Ayurveda. There are four states of Agni in Ayurveda, the following table gives the classification and the dosha responsible for the Agni state:

Dosha	Agni function	Sanskrit
All Doshas	Balanced	Sama
Vata	Variable / Irregular	Visama
Pitta	Strong / High	Tīksna
Kapha	Low / Constant	Manda

The idea of Agni is that it is a direct reflection on the metabolic functions. This means if your Agni is low your metabolism is operating at a reduced level (hypo) as compared to a healthy state. Or if your Agni is high (hyper) then your whole metabolism will reflect this increased functioning. *Note that all the constitutions have balanced Agni when healthy* and all of them have problems when unhealthy.

These are the descriptions of the imbalanced state of Jathara Agni:

High/excessive Agni (Tīksna Agni) – literally *"sharp/quick digestion"*.

When Jathara Agni is high, there is a regular, fast, strong metabolism. This creates a ravenous appetite that is capable of digesting large amounts of almost anything. This type of agni creates a digestion that "over cooks" the food and forms a poor quality of nutrients. High Agni usually results in several soft to loose bowel movements per day. If left untreated, digestive complaints involving heat and high acidity will manifest, such as acid reflux, or a burning feeling around the navel. High Agni is caused by excess Pitta Dosha.

Low/deficient Agni (Manda Agni) – literally *"dull/slow digestion"*.

When Agni is low, the metabolism is regular, slow and weak. There will be less hunger and it takes a long time to digest whatever has been eaten. In extreme cases even the most frugal meal can result in feelings of heaviness, indigestion and lead to constipation due to accumulation. If left unchecked, low Agni can result in excess mucus production responsible for feelings of nausea, heaviness, and congestion in general. Low Agni is caused by high or excess Kapha Dosha.

Variable Agni (Visama Agni) – literally *"variable digestion"*.

When Agni is variable, it is either too sharp/fast/strong or too dull/slow/weak. It is the only unstable form of Agni as the other states of Agni are regular. Appetite and digestion can be erratic, hence on one day you might be able to digest almost anything, whereas the next day digestion of a light meal is a problem. Variable Agni leads to abdominal bloating, excess gas and dry types of constipation. It can also lead to irritable bowel syndrome where diarrhoea and constipation alternate from one day to the next. Variable Agni is caused by high or excess Vata Dosha.

A large segment of the population suffers from poor assimilation of nutrients. This is the outcome of Agni being in any state other than "balanced" (Sama Agni). If assimilation is disturbed then all of the previous stages of digestion must be functioning poorly or incorrectly. When the body is not able to use and assimilate what it consumes then the body has to try and eliminate the undigested food somehow. Most of the undigested, or unused, material is eliminated from the body by the intestines. Unfortunately, if this becomes habitual then the undigested food begins to accumulate over time in the intestinal tract and putrefy. Rotting material in the intestinal tract puts an extra burden on the immune system and digestive organs. This is one of the major causes of degenerating diseases in the world. In Ayurveda the accumulation of undigested foods is directly related to the state of Agni function – if Agni is deranged the putrid material will manifest.

Ama – Non-Digested Food

When Jathara Agni is imbalanced it fails to digest food properly. The by-product of this poor digestion is Ama. Ama is the opposite of Agni, in other words when Agni is balanced it is impossible for Ama to be formed. The definition of Ama is:

"Food that has not been assimilated or evacuated is called Ama"

That substance which stays in the warm, dark, humid environment of the intestines begins to putrefy and rot. Ama does not have a supportive role in the body, in fact, it inhibits the body from functioning normally, eventually causing disease. Ama reduces our resistance to infection and encourages excessive levels of unhealthy bacteria and viruses because it reduces the capacity of Agni to function correctly. The more Ama we produce, the more it adheres to the tissue membranes, blocking communication and creating all manner of physiological imbalances. Ama can also include man-made pollutants, chemicals or any substance that comes into the body and is not assimilated as a nutrient or eliminated as a waste by the body.

The more Ama accumulates in our intestines, the more our digestion will be affected. Eventually, Ama will be absorbed into the bloodstream and circulate within the body. It will eventually find its way to some resting point – a weak spot in a Dhatu – where it will begin to accumulate. The main signs of Ama accumulation as it increases in the intestines and starts to overflow in the body's tissues are:

- **Fatigue, heaviness and tiredness** – The most common signs of Ama
- **Bad breath** – Rotting food in the G.I. tract
- **Headaches or migraines** – There are different causes of headaches and migraines, Ama is one of the most common
- **Tongue coating** – A whitish film you see on the surface of your tongue, especially when you get up in the morning indicate Ama in the intestines
- **Stool that sinks in the toilet** – non-digested food can also be seen in the stool
- **Chronic digestive problems** – are also a sign of Ama accumulation

Ama is produced when Jathara Agni becomes imbalanced. Remember that it is the three Doshas that control Agni function on all levels. If Agni is not working correctly and Ama is being formed the cause is one of the Doshas, not the Agni itself. Remember that Agni is controlled by Dosha.

One important point to understand about Ama is that it does not have legs! In other words Ama cannot move around the body without being attached to a Dosha. When this happens the Dosha can carry the Ama into the Dhatus and cause diseases in body. In Sanskrit the preface "SA" means "with". So when we add SA + ĀMA we get SĀMA. Be careful! SĀMA means "with toxins" and SAMA means "balanced". The long "A" changes completely the meaning of the word in Sanskrit. In Ayurveda there is a term for each Dosha mixed with Ama. These terms are as follows:

- Sāmavāta   = āma with Vāta
- SāmaPitta   = āma with Pitta
- Sāmakapha   = āma with Kapha

This concept is important because it means that Ama is never alone *outside* of the digestive system. Once Ama moves out of the intestines it is "hitchhiking" with a Dosha.

The Doshas and the Process of Digestion

Three stages of digestion exist in Ayurveda that correspond to the functioning of the three Doshas. These three steps of digestion are all controlled by the Dosha combining with Jathara Agni. The concept behind these three stages follows the natural transformation of food by each Dosha.

1. Kapha stage (liquefaction)

The first stage of digestion occurs in the mouth and stomach. It is dominated by Kapha and the Kapha secretions of the stomach. This allows the earth and water elements to be digested. It is the preliminary stage of digestion that renders the food liquid and homogenous and capable of being transformed by the digestive fire. Kapha controls mixing and liquefaction of the food. Most Kapha problems occur at this stage of digestion; like nausea, lack of appetite, heaviness, bloating and vomiting. This stage lasts from 1 to 2 hours.

2. Pitta stage (transformation and assimilation)

The second stage of digestion occurs at the end of the stomach and the beginning of the small intestine. It is dominated by Pitta and the Pitta secretions of the liver, gall bladder, pancreas and small intestine. In this stage food is transformed and releases heat and energy to the body. Pitta controls the transformation and assimilation of nutrients. This is the main location of Agni and where macro nutrient assimilation takes place. Most Pitta problems occur at this stage of digestion; like hyperacidity, heartburn and ulcers. This stage starts 2 hours after eating and lasts from 6 to 24 hours depending on the type of food eaten.

3. Vata stage (assimilation and elimination)

The third stage of digestion occurs at the colon. It is dominated by Vata and the Vata actions of movement and evacuation. At this stage Vata Dosha dries out the liquid food through the absorption of micro nutrients. The waste material – e.g., non-nutritive – that is left over is discarded as faeces. Vata controls assimilation and elimination in the stage. Most Vata problems occur at this stage of digestion; like bloating, distension, gas and constipation. This stage starts after the last stage ends and can last from 12 to 72 hours depending on the type of foods eaten.

The above information is needed in diagnosis and pathology and is introduced here as part of physiology because it is controlled by Dosha. The course will go deeper into this subject in the sections on diagnosis.

The Three Malas

This lesson looks closer at the waste products that are made by the function of Agni at all three levels (Jathara Agni, Panchabhuta Agni & Dhatva Agni). Basically, Mala, or waste products, are a normal function of metabolism and an important sign of health. Each level of Agni metabolism makes its own Mala that is removed and evacuated through the channels (Srotas) that exist for this purpose.

The three primary Malas and their corresponding elements are:

1. Feces (*purisha* - earth & water)
2. Urine (*mutra* - water & fire)
3. Sweat (*sveda* - fire & water)

The word "Mala" comes from the Sanskrit root "mal", to darken, stain or harm. Unlike Doshas they do not have a constructive function in the body. They do help to maintain body function by removing old, dead or non-usable matter.   Waste materials themselves can be damaged or vitiated by Dosha. The excess Doshas can affect them in a number of ways - mainly by mixing with them and carrying them to the Dhatus where they become lodged. When the Mala mix with Dosha the pathology becomes more difficult to treat; this subject will be explain in detail in one of the lessons on Pathology. There will also be a full discussion on the Malas in Diagnosis lessons as they allow us to judge the overall state of Dosha and Agni according to their nature.

In normal functions the body should eliminate the stool once per day in the morning. For people who eat an easy to digest diet - such as Vegetarian or Vegan - a second evacuation in the late morning or early afternoon can be normal. Urination should occur five to ten times a day depending on the amount of liquid consumed and lifestyle. Night urination usually shows a problem unless the lifestyle habits of drinking liquids before bed are in practice. Urination in the night can also be the secondary effect of medication. Sweating should occur during exercise, physical exertion or hot weather. If transpiration happens at other times it can indicate a problem of Meda Dhatu, Kapha Dosha, or a number of other factors. If the Malas show different patterns than indicated above, or as per the lifestyle habits, it may indicate abnormality of Agni, Dosha or Ama accumulation.

All three levels of the Agni metabolism are important. The Maha Malas (great or most important wastes) are the stool, urine and sweat. The Mala produced in the liver by the Panchabhuta Agni are mixed with liver bile and eliminated into the duodenum (first part of the small intestine). Mala that is produced by the Dhatva Agni in Dhatu metabolism are carried to either Rasa or Rakta Dhatu where they are cleaned by the liver and kidneys. Dhatu Mala is then removed either through stool or urine. Rasa and Rakta can also use the sweat channels (Sveda) to remove Mala. Thus, we see the importance of correct Dhatu metabolism and the Dhatva Agnis in keeping the body free of waste materials.

Purisha - feces or stool

The function of the feces is to give support (avasthamabhana) to the body and to anchor Vata Dosha. The stool helps to prevent organ prolapse by maintaining the tone of the colon, and the organs in the lower abdomen. The bulk of the stool is not actually food, but dead microorganisms that live in the colon and that are responsible to further transform nutrients after the Jathara Agni. Whatever earth element that is not assimilated also collects here.

Feces comes from the action of the Jathara Agni and serves to discharge excess earth and non-nutritive substances from the body

"Excess of feces causes abdominal enlargement, gurgling noises, pain and distention and a feeling of heaviness."
(AS.SU.11.12)

An excess of stool allows too much earth element in the body and increases the possibility of Ama formation. Feces alone will not indicated bad breath and body odor. These are signs of Ama accumulation and fermentation with the stool. When these combine it causes indigestion, headaches, dullness and constipation.

"Deficiency of feces causes movements of gas in the intestines, gurgling noises, and upwards movements of vayu to the heart and sides (flanks)."
(AS.SU.11.21)

A deficiency of stool allows a reduction of earth element in the body. This causes apana vayu to increase as there is less of the opposite element (earth) to hold it stable in the colon. When apana vayu accumulates it allows gas formation, noise in the colon, nervousness and the upward movement of the other forms of Vata in the body. This can cause chest pain, palpitations and lower back ache and general aches and pains in the body.

Purisha Mala is damaged by such factors as excess use of purgatives or colonics, by food that is too heavy or too light, by bad food combinations, by excess travel, by sleeping late, by coffee and drugs, by antibiotics, by dysentery, by inadequate exercise and by emotional factors such as worry and fear.

Mutra - urine

The function of urine is to eliminate soluble wastes. The kidneys extract the soluble wastes from the bloodstream, as well as excess water, sugars, and a variety of other compounds. Urine contains high concentrations of urea and other substances, including toxins that left over from digestive and Dhatu metabolism. All three forms of Agni are contributing to the waste products in urine.

Urine comes from the action of the kidneys and bladder (Mutravaha Srota) and is mainly under the control of Kapha with secondary support from Vata Dosha. The Mutra Mala is very important to remove excess Pitta and the fire element from the system.

"Excess of urine causes pain in the bladder and a feeling of needing to urinate even after having just finished urination."
(AS.SU.11.13)

Excess urine usually involves water retention (edema), frequent urination and thirst. It can show an excess of Kapha or a hypo-function of apana vayu. Mutra is directly related to Rasa, Rakta and Meda Dhatus - these tissues and their Doshas should be evaluated when there are indications of imbalance.

"Deficiency of urine causes small amounts of urine, difficult urination, discoloration of urine or blood in the urine."
(AS.SU.11.21)

Deficient urination can be related to Kapha and the Dhatus it controls. Pitta and Vata disorders can lower the water element and plasma (Rasa) in the body. Insufficient urination also allows toxins to accumulate in the liver and kidneys. These waste products are generally acidic or Pitta like in nature and can modify the pH of the plasma (Rasa and Rakta Dhatus).

Mutra Mala is damaged by use of diuretic drugs, the wrong herbs, the wrong foods, by drinking too much, by drinking too little, by alcohol, by excess sex, stress, and by emotional shock.

Sveda - sweat

The function of sweat is to eliminate soluble wastes through the skin. Sweat is a waste product of Meda Dhatu and allows the deeper tissues to remove toxins and waste products through a more direct route. Sweat also aids in the cooling of the body, although this not so much a function of the Mala as a function of Meda Dhatu.

Sweat comes from the action of Dhatva Agni. It allows the fire element, or Pitta like wastes, to be removed in a liquid form from the skin. Strong smelling sweat shows high Pitta or a Pitta constitution. In cases where Ama has moved into the deeper tissues sweat can also carry the odor of Ama mixed with a Dosha.

"Excess of sweat causes profuse sweating, unpleasant body odor and itching or irritation."
(AS.SU.11.14)

Excess sweating reduces Meda, Rasa and Rakta Dhatus in that order. As sweat removes heat (Pitta) from the body excess sweating can cause an increase in odor. Itching or irritation in the skin happens due to the increase of acid toxins or fire element being removed from through the skin.

"Deficiency of sweat causes absence of sweating, hair falling out, stiffness of the hair and cracking of the skin."
(AS.SU.11.22)

Deficient sweating shows a problem in Meda Dhatu. It is the Asthi Dhatu that is responsible for the production and maintenance of body hair. If Meda is incapable to nourish Asthi then symptoms relating to hair loss and dry hair result. Additionally, the skin is lubricated by Meda and dry, or cracking skin, indicate deficiency in Meda Dhatu.

Sevda Mala is damaged by the excessive use of diaphoretic herbs, sweating methods (saunas, jacuzzi, hammam, sweat lodges, etc.), by food that is too dry, by a lack of salt, and too much or too little exercise.

Conclusion

Remember that all the Malas can be modified by the primary or secondary effects of medications (allopathic or chemical).

Problems in the Malas show problems in Dosha, Dhatu and Agni. If the Mala are not eliminated on a daily basis it means that the body will become polluted by waste. This waste will mix with Dosha and be transported into the Dhatus. The correct use of Malas is to develop the habit of observing them on a daily basis. As practitioners this habit needs to be taught to the patients. The more the patient becomes involved in the observation of their own Mala the more they can see the changes they make in diet and lifestyle. They also become responsible for following the evolution of their health.

Study Questions for Chapter Seven

1. What is the difference between Agni and Pitta Dosha?

2. What is the primary difference between Agni and Ama?

3. What are the names of the three groups of Agni?

4. Which form of Agni is most important for health?

5. Agni relates to enzyme function on a physical level. What is an enzyme?

6. Which state of Agni does not create Ama?

7. What is Mala?

8. How do Mala create disease?

9. Mala acts like Ama under what circumstances?

10. Problems with the Malas show problems in which part of the anatomy?

CHAPTER EIGHT
THE SROTAMSI

After the three Doshas there are four primary divisions in Ayurvedic anatomy – Dhatu (tissues), Srotamsi (channels), Mala (waste products) and Kalas (membranes that define and separate). Central to Ayurveda is the channel system (Srotamsi) through which the Dosha move and communicate with the organism. These channel systems are also responsible for nourishing the Dhatu of the body through receiving and distributing outside substances. Examples of this would be food, water, air, sunlight and heat. When the Srotamsi function correctly they allow the normal metabolism of food, liquid, air and sunlight throughout the body.

The Srotamsi are called *Srotas* when spoken of individually and when plural are called *Srotamsi*. As a functional system of medicine Ayurveda is very concerned with the systems or channels that allow the movement and communication between Dosha and Dhatu. The Srota are often not listed as separate from Dhatu in Ayurveda. In the *Asthanga Hrdayam*, Sharirasthana section, Chapter 3, Sutra 40 there is a clear distinction from those Srota that communicate with the outside - nine of them - and those listed in Sutra 41 - thirteen of them. The classic manner of explaining the Srotamsi is illustrated in the following manner:

Bāhya Srotas (channels that lead to external orifices)

These Srotas are nine in number for men and twelve in number for women.
2 - in the two nasal passages
2 - in the two ears
2 - in the two eyes
1 - mouth
1 - rectum
1 - urethra

There are three for women:
2 - breast milk passages
1 - menstruation passage

The Bāhya Srotas relate to three of the sense organs and three of the motor organs. These channels are considered large, or wide in size, and open to the exterior of the body through an opening. They are also called the nine doors of the body. They allow a connection of a specific place or organ to the outside world. They are not complex in nature generally and tend to indicate one function only; e.g. seeing, hearing, etc.

Abhyantra Srotas (channels that are mainly internal)

These Srotas are said to the seats of life, or places that have essential activities needed for the continued existence of life. There are thirteen of them.

1 - for Prana (respiration and metabolism of oxygen)
1 - for water metabolism
1 - for food metabolism
7 - for Dhatu
3 - for Mala

These Srotas are very complex in function and physiology. They have multiple functions and locations. They are mainly internal even though six of these channels communicate with the outside world their primary functions are internal. Most modern books on Ayurveda (Western) combine the Bahya Srotas with the Abhyantra Srotas.

There are some important considerations to be made in understanding the difference between these two classifications. The first is that Bahya Srotas are basically simple in function and have one main action. The second is that the Abhyantra Srotas are complex and have a multitude of functions and locations. They are more like networks or systems than "channels". The third point is that the Abhyantra Srotas often are sites of metabolic activity - of physiological functioning and transformation of material. They are not simple channels that communicate with specific locations or that have single actions; for example, the two breasts and their channels carry milk to the baby. These channels have no other function. In this example be careful not confuse the nerve channels in the skin and nipples that allow for feeling and sensations - this is a Abhyantra Srotas, the Majjavaha Srotas.

From a modern point of view I think we can divide the Srotamsi into two main categories of Communication and Metabolism. The Bahya Srotas that allow the function of the three sense organs are not covered in this lesson because their function is simple and allows the sense organ to work. They do not need further explanations.

Srotamsi in Communication

The channels are the means of intelligent communication for the organism as a whole. They link not only all of the metabolic functions, but also the psychology to the physiology. They provide pathways for *physical* and *non-physical* communication. In other words communication can be the transportation of a physical substance or the transportation of a feeling.

It is important to realize that the Dhatus, or tissues, are the places where disease becomes installed, or located. However, the 'disease' needs first to arrive there, and second, needs to be nourished once it has taken up residency in the Dhatu. It is the Srotas that provide both these functions. Additionally, the organs are part of Dhatu and are subservient to the channel systems that both feed them and remove their waste materials. Treating the organs alone will never cure the disease totally because the Dhatu and Srota that support the organ must be healed or corrected first.

Through the Srota the Dhatu are nourished and strengthened. The waste materials (Malas) are eliminated through their own channels. The Mala Srotamsi only work efficiently when the other channels are functioning correctly. The supportive membranes (Kalas) are nourished and cleaned by the proper functioning of the Dhatus which are maintained by the channels. Thus the Srota support Dhatu, Mala and Kalā through the action of communication and transportation.

Srotamsi in Metabolism

The second major function of the channel system is that of controlling or facilitating metabolism. This idea is that a Srota is more than just a tube that connects one place to another place. Many Srota are actually networks of collective "systems" and not "tubes". When we begin to look at the Srotas more from the point of view of collective systems it is possible to understand their role in metabolizing substances.

A modern definition of metabolism is:

"Metabolism is the set of chemical reactions that happen in living organisms to maintain life. These *processes* allow organisms to grow and reproduce, maintain their structures, and respond to their environments. The chemical reactions of metabolism are organized into metabolic *pathways*, in which one chemical is transformed through a series of steps into another chemical.

The metabolism of an organism determines which substances it will find nutritious and which it will find poisonous. The speed of metabolism, the metabolic rate, also influences how much food an organism will require. A striking feature of metabolism is the similarity of the basic metabolic *pathways* and components between even vastly different species. These striking similarities in metabolism are probably due to the high efficiency of these *pathways*, and their early appearance in evolutionary history."

This modern definition of metabolism could almost be an Ayurvedic description. Note the italics I added into the text above. Modern medicine first describes metabolism as a number of *processes* in the body. Next it has to use the word "pathways" to allow for the metabolic processes that are continuously taking place in the body.

It is important to understand that the Srotamsi systems are these same systems that allow metabolic processes to take place in the body. Therefore, the Srotas that allows us to breath - Pranavaha Srotas - is more than just a tube that allows air into and out of the body. It is a system that metabolizes the air we breathe into our body. Yes, it brings it into and out the body, and it allows the chemical processes that receive the nutrients that sustain our lives. Yet, it also extracts Prana from the breath and assimilates it into the body.

Most people are now classifying the Srotas into fourteen systems because they add the channel of the mind into the classification of the thirteen Abhyantra Srotas. For women we take the two Srotas from the Bāhya Srotas classification to give sixteen total.

There are sixteen main Srotamsi:

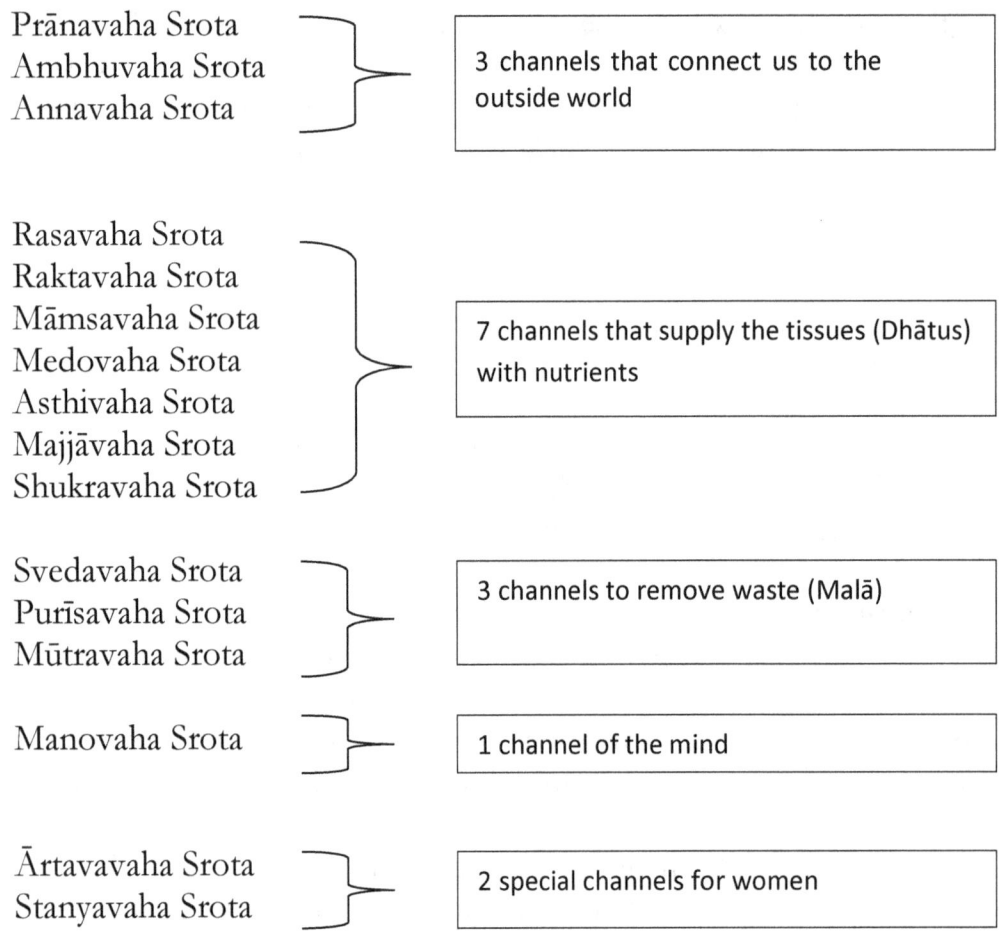

Prānavaha Srota
Ambhuvaha Srota
Annavaha Srota

3 channels that connect us to the outside world

Rasavaha Srota
Raktavaha Srota
Māmsavaha Srota
Medovaha Srota
Asthivaha Srota
Majjāvaha Srota
Shukravaha Srota

7 channels that supply the tissues (Dhātus) with nutrients

Svedavaha Srota
Purīsavaha Srota
Mūtravaha Srota

3 channels to remove waste (Malā)

Manovaha Srota

1 channel of the mind

Ārtavavaha Srota
Stanyavaha Srota

2 special channels for women

Description of the 16 Main Channels

The following three channels bring nourishment into the body:

1) PRĀNAVAHASROTA (breath metabolism)

This is the most important channel as it carries the 'life force' or Prāna into the body. It includes the absorption and distribution of air (oxygen) and includes breathing and the respiration system. This Srotas controls the metabolism of breathing. If this system breaks down we die very quickly as it provides the primary source of life for our bodies.

The Prānavaha Srotas is not limited to the physical channels as it includes the Nādī system of Yoga as well (72,000 nādīs). It is primarily through the Prānavaha Srotas that the five forms of Vata (the 5 Vayus) move and control the whole body. This Srotas also joins the physical body with the Prānamayakosha (energetic envelope) and through this *envelope* links the physical to the mental. This Srotas is mainly the domain of Vata Dosha from a functional point of view.

2) AMBHUVAHASROTA (liquid metabolism)

This is the network of systems that coordinates the water metabolism in the body. It has a broader definition than in modern anatomy as it links kidney function with pancreas functions to digest and regulate fats and simple sugar in the fluid of plasma and blood (Rasa Dhatu). After the Prānavaha Srotas this is the one of the most important channels. It allows the body to be hydrated and lubricated. It helps to cool and maintain body heat. This system allows the body to receive liquids from the outside and to metabolize them until they become part of the body. This Srotas is mainly the domain of Kapha Dosha from a functional point of view.

3) ANNAVAHASROTA (food metabolism)

This is the channel that carries food – the digestive tract. Most disease starts from a poorly functioning digestive system. This channel is also called the *Koshta* as it holds the three Dosha. After the Prānavaha Srotas this is the one of the most important channels. This Srotas is responsible for the metabolism of food and all matter taken into the body. It is a complex series of systems that include different Dhatus and organs. This system is involved in almost all forms of disease and pathology. This Srotas is mainly the domain of Pitta Dosha from a functional point of view.

The following seven channels serve the seven Dhatus:

4) RASAVAHASROTA (fluid metabolism)

Rasavaha relates to plasma fluid circulation in the blood and the lymphatic system. This system works closely with the Ambhuvaha Srotas to control all fluids in the body. This system takes the fluids that have been metabolized by Ambhuvaha Srotas and uses them to control primary fluid metabolism. Because of this important role it supports all other Dhatu and Srotamsi.

5) RAKTAVAHASROTA (blood metabolism)

This is the channel that relates directly to the red blood cell circulation which carries and circulates heat, oxygen and nutrients throughout the body. It is responsible to remove waste products from the blood and works closely with several organs, glands and Dhatus. This is also one of the main travel routes for the three Doshas in the body because it needs to irrigate every cell in the body. So while Rakta Dhatu is the production and maintenance of red blood cells - Raktavaha Srotas is the circulation of these red blood cells with their nutrients and chemicals.

6) MĀMSAVAHASROTA (muscle metabolism)

This is the system that nourishes the muscle tissues. This metabolism of nutrients allows for the formation of Mamsa Dhatu. Mamsavaha Srotas is quite vast and includes a number of small to large channels. These channels also remove the waste products generated by movement, exercise and metabolism of muscle tissue.

7) MEDOVAHASROTA (fat metabolism)

This is the system that nourishes the fat tissues. This metabolism of nutrients allows for the formation of Meda Dhatu. These channels also remove the waste products generated by movement, exercise and metabolism of fat tissue. This system is linked to the kidney function that cleans and adds lipid matter into our plasma.

8) ASTHIVAHASROTA (bone metabolism)

This is the system that nourishes the bone tissues. This metabolism of nutrients allows for the formation of Asthi Dhatu. These channels also remove the waste products generated by the metabolism of bone tissue.

9) MAJJĀVAHASROTA (marrow and nerve metabolism)

This is the system that nourishes the bone marrow and nerve tissues and removes waste products associated with normal metabolism. This system has a dual role as it also allows for primary communication in the body. It allows the movement of Vata Dosha in the body. It is Vata Dosha that provides the basic impulse of nerve movement. This Srotas has two major actions: 1) support, nourish and remove waste from the tissue, and 2) allow basic communications to take place all over the body.

Often the function of communication is confused with the Majja Dhatu. The Dhatu provides the basic physical structure and the Srotas provides the means to move nerve impulses within this structure. This Srotas works closely with the Prānavaha Srotas.

10) SHUKRAVAHASROTA (reproductive metabolism)

This is the system that nourishes the reproductive tissues and removes the waste products associated with normal metabolism. The metabolism of nutrients in this Dhatu allows for the formation of Ojas.

The following three channels remove waste from the body:

11) SVEDAVAHASROTA (waste channel)

The system that removes liquid waste and toxins through sweat. It also allows a cleansing action that removes dirt and waste from the skin. This system helps to clean Rasa, Rakta and Meda Dhatus.

12) PURĪSAVAHASROTA (waste channel)

The system that removes solid waste and toxins through the stool. This system is more complex than the Bāhya Srotas of the rectum. This channel includes all of the Large Intestine (colon) and allows for a number of important processes. For example, if this system is too fast the liquid in the stool will not have time to be absorbed and it is this liquid which carries the micro nutrients needed to nourish the body.

13) MŪTRAVAHASROTA (waste channel)

The system that removes liquid waste and toxins through urine. The removal of liquid waste from the body keeps all tissues clean. This system is linked to Rasa, Rakta and Meda Dhatus. It is also closely related to the correct function of Ambhuvaha Srotas.

The following channel allows the movement of thoughts:

14) MANOVAHASROTA (thinking and emotions metabolism)

This is the system of the mind, thinking, emotions, feelings and psychological aspects move through this channel. This system will be covered in a several other lessons on psychology. It is the Prāna vayu that allows this system to function.

The next two systems are only for women:

15) ĀRTAVAHASROTA (female menstrual system)

This system controls the menstrual fluid and is dependent on Rasadhatu and Raktadhatu. It is a complex system that removes waste products from the reproductive system and organs. The reproductive organs (uterus and vagina) are controlled by Pitta Dosha (see the lesson on organs and glands). Therefore, when the Upadhatu of Rasa meets with the Pitta organs - in other words Raktadhatu - it takes on the color and qualities of this Dhatu.

16) STANYAVAHASROTA (female lactation system)

This system controls lactation for new mothers and is dependent on Ārtavavahasrota (fluid and metabolism), Rasadhatu (fluid) and Shukradhatu (hormones).

In conclusion the Srotamsi are a sub-classification of Dhatu because their structure and form are made and maintained by Dhatu. From a functional point of view they are an independent part of anatomy - most specifically the physiological function of metabolism in the body.

The treatment of the channel systems is one of the primary objectives of all Ayurvedic therapies because they allow Dosha function, Dhatu metabolism and the removal of Mala. In Ayurveda the three Doshas are used to diagnose the patient and provide a model for therapeutic protocol. Then we use the "Twenty Attributes" or twenty Gunas to choose our therapeutic substances. However, it is the channel system that we actually address when using therapeutic substances – the Srotamsi are the physical destination of any treatment. This is because they provide the network of both communication, nourishment and metabolism in the human body. Through them we modify Dhatu construction and maintenance.

A last fundamental concept in Ayurveda is that heat opens the channels and cold contracts the channels. This is both on an external level (applying heat to the skin) and on an internal level (administering heating / cooling herbs or foods). To work internally we use substances that either open (those with heating qualities) or contract (those with cooling qualities) the channels. This is why the main classification of herbs after the effect on Doshas is that of heating or cooling (this is called *Vīrya* in Sanskrit). Basically if you want to open, clear, remove, stimulate or accelerate use heating substances. These will effectively open and clean the channels. However, if you wish to increase, build, close, sedate or calm use cooling substances. These are general rules on how any substance affects the body's systems.

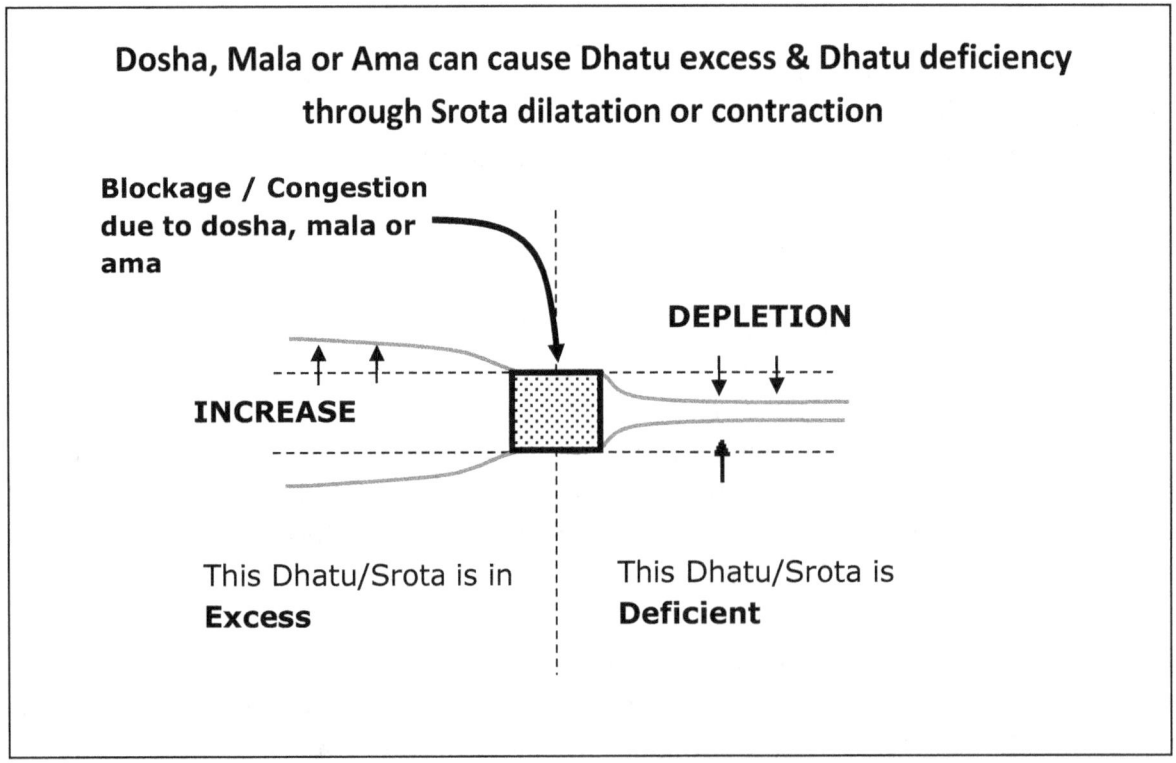

There are many different kinds of pathologies that can cause problems in the Srotamsi. This subject we will discuss in detail later in the course. The information in this chapter needs to be memorized.

Study Questions for Chapter Eight

1.   Why are the Srotamsi listed as part of the Dhatu in Ayurveda?

2.   The Asthanga Hridayam, Sharirasthana section states that there are two main kinds of Srota; what are they?

3.   Srota have two main functions in the body; what are they?

4.   What is communication between Dhatu controlled by?

5.   What are the membranes (Kalas) nourished and cleaned by?

6.   The Pranavaha Srotas is more than a tube; what is it?

7.   Why are there are sixteen Srota used today in Ayurveda?

8.   After the Pranavaha Srotas this is the most important Srotas; which Srotas is it?

9.   The Majjavaha Srotas allows the movement of Vata Dosha in the body. This Srotas has two major actions; what are they?

10.   Why is the treatment of the channel systems is one of the primary objectives of all Ayurvedic therapies?

CHAPTER NINE
THE ORGANS/GLANDS & DOSHA

In the Ayurvedic system emphasis is placed on the Dosha, Dhatus and Srotamsi. The organs and glands are part of the seven Dhatus in Ayurveda because the Dhatus manufacture and support the organs and glands. In classical Ayurveda the organs are given names and locations. They are important and recognized as having vital functions in the body. However, their health is dependent on the correct metabolic functioning of Dhatu and Srota of which they are part of and not independent from.

Organs/Glands and the Dhatu Correspondence

Rasa Dhatu is responsible for the manufacturing and maintenance of the lungs, stomach and mucus membranes. In general Rasa Dhatu is responsible for all organs and glands as it is controlling the fabrication and maintenance of all the following Dhatus.

Rakta Dhatu is responsible for the manufacturing and maintenance of the heart, liver, uterus/vagina, gall bladder and spleen. There are secondary actions to support the fabrication of the pancreas.

Mamsa Dhatu is responsible for the manufacturing and maintenance for the structure of all organs and glands. This means the walls, connective tissues, form and structure of all organs and glands are controlled by Mamsa Dhatu. Mamsa provides the rigidity, protection and structure to all organs and glands, just as it does to the whole body.

Meda Dhatu is responsible for the manufacturing and maintenance of the kidneys and in a secondary, supporting function to the pancreas, liver, adrenals and testes.

Asthi Dhatu is responsible for the manufacturing and maintenance of the bones and does not relate directly to the maintenance of any organ or gland.

Majja Dhatu is responsible for the manufacturing and maintenance of the brain and endocrine glands that are metabolic in function (hypothalamus, pituitary, pineal, thyroid, pancreas, and adrenal).

111

Shukra Dhatu is responsible for the manufacturing and maintenance of the endocrine glands that are growth related (hypothalamus, pituitary, thymus, testes and ovaries).

Organs/Glands and Srotamsi Correspondence

The Srotamsi can relate to the organs and glands in the following manner:
   1. **Pranavaha Srotas**, the respiratory system, relates to the lungs and heart.
   2. **Annavaha Srotas**, the digestive system, relates to the stomach, small intestine and colon.
   3. **Ambhuvaha Srotas**, the water metabolism system, relates to the pancreas and the kidneys, and secondarily to the urinary bladder.
   4. **Rasavaha Srotas**, the plasma circulation and lymphatic system, relates specifically to the liver, lungs, stomach and in general all organs and glands.
   5. **Raktavaha Srotas**, the red blood circulatory system, relates to the liver, spleen and heart, and secondarily to any organ or gland that holds heat.
   6. **Mamsavaha Srotas**, the muscular system, relates to the structural aspect of all organs and glands.
   7. **Medovaha Srotas**, the adipose system, relates to the kidneys.
   8. **Asthivaha Srotas**, the skeletal system, relates to the colon.
   9. **Majjavaha Srotas**, the nervous system, relates to the brain and endocrine glands.
   10. **Shukravaha Srotas**, the reproductive system, relates to the endocrine glands.
   11. **Svedavaha Srotas**, the sebaceous system, relates to the lungs.
   12. **Purishavaha Srotas**, the excretory system, relates to the colon.
   13. **Mutravaha Srotas**, the urinary system, relates to the bladder and kidneys.
   14. **Artavavaha Srotas**, the menstrual system, relates to the uterus, and secondarily to the liver.
   15. **Stanyavaha Srotas**, the lactation system, relates to the breasts and the endocrine glands of Shukra dhatu.
   16. **Manovaha Srotas**, the mental metabolism, relates to the brain and heart

Organs/Glands and the three Dosha Correspondence

The Doshas can relate to the organs and glands in the following manner:
   Vata   colon, urinary bladder, kidney, brain
   Pitta   small intestine, liver, gall bladder, spleen, heart, uterus
   Kapha   stomach, lungs, pancreas, testes

In general:
   Vata governs the function of all the organs.
   Pitta governs the metabolism in all organs.
   Kapha lubricates and maintains the structure of all organs.

Organs/Glands and their Functions

Here is a review of the organs by their functions and structure.

STOMACH (*amashaya*)

The stomach is a Kapha organ. It is the Mulasthana of Kapha and its main site of accumulation. Much of the body's phlegm is produced here. The stomach produces mainly Kapha fluids, like the various alkaline secretions of the stomach membrane. The main role of the stomach is to receive the solid food, liquefy it, and then mix it with any liquids that have been consumed. This should result in a thick liquid food mass that is transferred to the small intestines.

The stomach is damaged by wrong eating habits including overeating or underrating, bad food combinations, food that is too strong in taste, food that is too hot or too cold, or eating another meal before the previous one has left the stomach.

The stomach is linked to the mind and emotions through the Kapha Srotas systems. It is sensitive and can be affected by emotional factors, like worry and greed. The stomach manifests its aggravation as nausea, belching, vomiting, lack of appetite and indigestion – all showing an excess of Kapha.

SMALL INTESTINE (*garhani*)

The small intestine is a Pitta organ. It is the Mulasthana of Pitta and is the place where Pitta accumulates. It is also the main site of the digestive fire (Jathar Agni) and it produces mainly hot, acidic secretions. The primary role of the small intestine is to receive the liquid food mass from the stomach and subject it to strong digestive bile's (Agni) to extract the nutritive substances from the non-nutritive substances. After this has been accomplished in the first part of the small intestine (duodenum) the macro-nutrients in the food mass are assimilated in the remaining part of the small intestine. The small intestine is a major site of nutrient absorption.

The small intestine is damaged mainly by food that is too hot, spicy, sour or oily. It is deranged by stimulants like coffee and chocolate. All forms of alcohol cause problems here.

The small intestine is linked to mind and emotions through the Pitta Srotas systems. Mentally it is damaged by emotions such as irritability and anger. Its aggravation manifests as heartburn, hyperacidity or ulcers – all showing an excess of Pitta.

LARGE INTESTINE (*pakvashaya*)

The large intestine or colon is a Vata organ. It is the Mulasthana of Vata and is the site where Vata accumulates. Its purpose is to absorb the liquid from the food that has been produced by the stomach and refined by the small intestine. The large intestine is the major site of micro-nutrient absorption. When the liquid matter has been absorbed the remaining solid wastes are evacuated. There are special channels that communicate from the colon to the liver – these transport the micro-nutrients directly to the liver for the second stage of digestion.

The colon is damaged by food that is too cold, astringent, dry, light, or insufficient in bulk. It is also disturbed by the excessive use of laxatives, enemas or colonics.

The colon is linked to the mind and emotions through the Vata Srotas systems. Emotionally it is upset by stress, anxiety and fear. Its aggravation manifests as gas, distention and constipation – all showing an excess of Vata.

LUNGS (*kloman*)

The lungs, which are the basis for the respiratory system, are primarily a Kapha organ by structure and a Vata organ by function. Kapha keeps them lubricated and hydrated while Vata brings in nutrients and removes waste through respiration. The lungs are linked to Pranavaha Srotas and Rasavaha Srotas. They allow Prana and oxygen to absorbed from the air outside. Due to the hydration provided by Kapha these subtle nutrients can be absorbed into the Srotamsi. Because of the constant movement of the lungs the absorption of Prana and oxygen is possible. This constant movement requires a steady production of Kapha lubrication fluids to correctly maintain their normal function and to fix the absorbed Prana into the body.

The lungs are damaged by excessive exposure to cold, dampness and other environmental factors like heat or dryness. The inhalation of smoke, dust, air pollution or other air-born matter weakens the lungs.

The lungs are linked to both the Kapha and Vata Srotamsi. They are emotionally sensitive, receptive and easily damaged. They are harmed by grief and sorrow due to Kapha emotions. Vata dries them out and related to Vata emotions like stress, fear and anxiety. Their aggravation appears as phlegm, cough, asthma and difficult breathing.

HEART (*hrdaya*)

The heart is a Pitta organ by function and a Kapha organ by structure. It is linked to both Rakta dhatu and Raktavaha Srotas for the circulation of plasma (Rasa) and red blood cells (Rakta). So even in function Kapha is closely related to this organ. The heart circulates the nutrients absorbed by lungs in the form of both Rasa and Rakta. Because of the constant movement of the heart every cell in the body is nourished with Prana and oxygen. This constant movement requires a steady production of Kapha lubrication fluids to correctly maintain the hearts normal function as a pump.

The heart is damaged by many of the same things that damage the small intestine as it is a Pitta organ. Oils, fats and alcohol are the most damaging foods. Lifestyle habits like overwork, or over exercise, or no work, no exercise are also damaging.

The heart is linked to the Vata Srotamsi as Vata controls the nerve plexus that allow the heart to beat. Thus, emotionally, the heart is mainly disturbed by excessive Vata emotions – either positive or negative. It is damaged by any emotional trauma and/or the suppression of emotions. The heart manifests disorders as palpitations, high or low blood pressure, arrhythmia, heart pains and any circulatory problem. For the circulation it is linked to Raktavaha Srotas and manifests it's Pitta attributes here.

LIVER (*yakrt*)

The liver, which is involved with both the digestive and circulatory systems, is primarily a Pitta gland, and secondarily a Kapha gland. The liver is responsible for cleansing and removing toxins from the blood. It also regulates hormone levels in the blood. It is the most important place of bile production (Agni) and is also the site of the second stage of digestion (5 bhuta Agni). The liver works closely with the small intestine to control the digestive process. The liver also has a very close relation to the pancreas and can take over most of the pancreases bile production if needed. It is involved with sugar and fat metabolism along with the pancreas.

The liver is damaged by Pitta increasing factors like too much spicy, greasy, or sweet food. Also an excess of alcohol and drugs damage it. There may be a bitter taste in the mouth or acid burps when the liver is deranged.

The liver is linked mainly to the Pitta Srotas and reflects the Pitta emotions when disrupted.

GALL BLADDER (part of liver so – *yakrt*)

The Gall Bladder is primarily a Pitta organ. It is considered to be a part of the liver as it holds the digestive bile and secrets it when needed. Basically it has the same qualities as the liver, except that the livers role is very complex and the gall bladder has only one role – releasing bile.

All factors that derange the liver harm the gall bladder. Note that the gall bladder is often damaged before the liver and shows imbalances in the liver long before the liver is diseased. The most common problems are stones or accumulation of calcified bile in the gall bladder or it ducts.

The gall bladder is linked mainly to the Pitta Srotas and reflects the Pitta emotions when disrupted.

PANCREAS (also called – *kloman*)

The pancreas is primarily a Kapha gland and secondarily a Pitta gland. It is unique in that it is both an endocrine and exocrine gland. It relates closely to the liver and can take over some of the livers digestive functions if needed. The pancreas controls sugar and fat metabolism that relate to the Ambhuvaha Srotas. It also assists in bile production and secretion into the small intestine.

The pancreas is damaged by eating too much sweet, rich food, and by drinking carbonated drinks. Any kind of synthetic drink (colas, energy drinks, etc.) damage this gland very quickly and cause diabetes among other disease.

The pancreas is linked to the Kapha Srotas system and relates mainly to Kapha type emotional factors. Some of its dysfunction manifests as irregular sugar metabolism; hypoglycemia and diabetes.

SPLEEN (*pliha*)

The spleen is primarily a Pitta organ. It is involved with recycling iron, blood formation and destruction. It is the emergency storage location for blood. If there is a sudden blood loss the spleen releases blood to protect the body. It is also involved with the immune system through retaining white blood cells (Monocytes). The spleen synthesizes antibodies in its white pulp and removes antibody-coated bacteria along with antibody-coated blood cells by way of blood and lymph node circulation. The spleen is part of the lymphatic system according to modern medicine. In Ayurveda is relates to both Rakta and Rasa dhatus.

The spleen is damaged by most of the same factors as the liver and by traumatic injuries. As it is part of Rasa dhatu it is also damaged by the same factor that damage Rasa dhatu.

The spleen is linked mainly to the Pitta Srotas and reflects the Pitta emotions when disrupted.

KIDNEYS (*vrkkau*)

The kidneys are primarily Vata organs and secondary Kapha. The kidneys are paired organs with several functions. They are organs of elimination for the water element and by removing the uric acid from the blood, aid in cleansing it and removing excess Pitta. The kidneys excrete wastes such as urea and ammonium. They are also responsible for the re-absorption of water, glucose, and amino acids. The kidneys also produce important hormones including calcitriol and rennin (absorption of calcium and regulating blood pressure, etc.).

The kidneys are damaged by too much travel, exposure to cold, excessive sex, and psychological trauma; they are sensitive organs. They link to the Ambhuvaha Srotas and are involved in most disorders of lymph and water (edema, etc.). They are also linked to Medovaha Srotas for nourishment and support.

Psychologically the kidneys are damaged by Vata emotions like fear and fright; and Kapha emotions such as greed and stinginess.

URINARY BLADDER (*basti*)

The urinary bladder is primarily a Vata organ. It is the organ that releases urine when needed. Ayurveda considers it to be a vital organ for life. It is considered to be an extension of the kidneys and all the indications for the kidney apply to great extent to the bladder. Note that the bladder – like the gall bladder – has only one simple role; to release urine. The kidneys have a complex role.

The urinary bladder is damaged by too much sex, suppression of the urge to urinate or diet that is too acidic in nature. Its dysfunction manifests as difficult urination, abnormal urination, burning urination and lower back pain.

Psychologically the bladder is damaged by Vata emotions like fear and fright.

BRAIN (*sadhaka* or *murdha*)
The brain is primarily a Vata organ as it is the source of the nerve impulses that govern the rest of the body. The cerebrospinal fluid is Kapha in nature (Tarpaka Kapha) and it serves to support the Vata function of the brain and nerves (Majja dhatu). Without the proper Kapha in the brain, Vata will accumulate.

The brain is damaged by external factors in the form of excess sensory stimuli. Other factors include excessive use of stimulants like coffee, alcohol or drugs (prescription or recreational). Internal factors include too much thought, worry or stress. Derangement of the brain manifests as insomnia, hallucinations, spasms, tremors, paralysis, etc.

REPRODUCTIVE ORGANS (testicles – *Vrsana*; Ovaries – *Artava*; uterus – *Yoni*)
The male reproductive glands, testes, are primarily Kapha glands. The female reproductive glands, ovaries, are also primarily Kapha glands. The female system is more complex than the male system, which is simply the production and ejaculation of sperm. The uterus is primarily a Pitta organ because it is part of Rakta dhatu. Therefore, the uterus and vagina are fiery in nature whereas the penis is watery in nature; this creates a polarity of opposites.

The menstrual fluid is the upadhatu of Rasa dhatu. When it is brought to the uterus by the Artavavaha Srotas it takes on the Pitta attributes of the uterus. This gives the fluid a reddish color. The vagina is considered to be a part of the uterus, so both are under the control of Rakta dhatu and Pitta dosha.

The sperm and ovum are controlled by Kapha dosha as they are the root of all structure in a new born child. They allow growth and form to manifest. Hence, the endocrine aspect is Kapha in nature and reproduction is a Kapha function when fertility is concerned. Vata dosha controls the cycles of time and coordinates the other two doshas in their functions in the reproductive system.

The reproductive organs are damaged by too much sex, repression of sex, by poor nutrition, stress and by strong emotions. Their aggravation manifests as impotence, infertility; mainly Vata disorders.

Psychologically the reproductive system relates to all three doshas.

Endocrine system as per Ayurveda

Here is an explanation of the Endocrine system as per Ayurveda. It was already explained under the Dhatu section of this lesson that this system is controlled by Majja and Shukra Dhatu's. Majja is controlling the development of the metabolic endocrine glands and Shukra controls the growth hormones that include sexual functions.

Endocrine Gland and Hormone Secreted / controlling Dosha	Functions	Sub-Dosha Relation by function
1. **Hypothalamus** - release factors for STH, TSH, FSH, LH, PRL, ACTH, MSH that are secreted from the pituitary, and secrets Vasopressin and Oxytocin to the pituitary. / all 3 doshas	Stimulates the secretion and release of pituitary hormones, inhibits these same hormones from being secreted, Vasopressin & Oxytocin are made here.	**Vata** - Prana Vayu **Pitta** - Sadhaka Pitta **Kapha** - Tarpaka Kapha is not directly related yet it provides the cerebral fluid in which the brain functions.
2. **Pituitary** - Somatotropin (STH), Thyrotropin (TSH), Follicle Stimulating (FSH), Luteinizing (LH), Prolactin (PRL), Adrenocorticotropin (ACTH), Melancyte Stimulating (MSH), Vasopressin (ADH), Oxytocin / all 3 dosha	Releases all the hormones given on the left to regulate metabolism, growth, protein synthesis, the thyroid gland, controls ovaries & testes, estrogen's & progesterone's, lactation, adrenal function, blood pressure, kidney function.	Same as above.
3. **Pineal** - Melatonin (MLT), Serotonin / Vata dosha	Influences cyclic activities in metabolism and sexual maturity; functions are not completely understood	**Vata** - Prana Vayu

4. **Thyroid** - Thyroxine, Calcitonin /Pitta dosha	Regulates basal metabolism, growth & development.	**Vata** - Udana Vayu **Pitta** - Pachaka and Sadhaka Pitta
5. **Parathyroid** - Parathyroid Hormone / Pitta dosha	Regulates the blood level of calcium & phosphorus	**Vata** - Udana Vayu **Pitta** - Ranjaka Pitta
6. **Thymus** - Thymosin, Thymopoietin, others /Kapha dosha	Influences the lymphatic glands, general immunity, cell immunity through production of T-cells and growth, functions are not completely understood.	**Vata** - Prana Vayu, Vyana Vayu **Kapha** - Avalambaka Kapha
7. **Adrenal** - Glucocorticoids (DHEA and others), Mineralocorticoids, estrogens, progesterones, androgens, testosterone / Vata dosha, Kapha 2nd	Influences carbohydrate, protein, & fat metabolism; anti-inflammatory & immunosuppressive; regulates sodium, potassium & water metabolism in general; supplements the action of the ovaries & testes.	**Vata** - Samana Vayu, Apana Vayu **Pitta** - Pachaka Pitta **Kapha** - Kledaka Kapha
8. **Pancreas** - Insulin, Glucagon /Kapha dosha, Pitta 2nd	Helps utilize glucose, regulates blood sugar through the secretion of these two hormones which are opposite in action to each other.	**Vata** - Samana Vayu, **Pitta** - Pachaka Pitta, **Kapha** - Kledaka Kapha
9. **Ovaries** - Estrogen's, Progesterone's, Relxin / Kapha dosha, Pitta and Vata 2nd	Regulates the development of female sexual organs, fertility, controls menstruation with FSH & LH, relaxes pelvic muscles and ligaments.	**Vata** - Apana Vayu **Pitta** - Ranjaka Pitta & secondary Pachaka Pitta **Kapha** - Tarpaka Kapha
10. **Testes** - Testosterone, Estradiol, etc. / Kapha dosha, Pitta and Vata 2nd	In men, testosterone regulates the development of male reproductive tissues such as the testis and prostate as well as promoting secondary sexual characteristics such as increased muscle, bone mass and hair growth.	**Vata** - Apana Vayu **Pitta** - Ranjaka Pitta & secondary Pachaka Pitta **Kapha** - Tarpaka Kapha

These are the main endocrine glands. Note that there are other glands or systems that produce hormones.

The Seven Kalas /Membranes

Each of the seven Dhatu and their corresponding Srotas has a number of membranes that allow for the absorption and diffusion of nutrients. These membranes serve to demarcate the underlying tissue from its channels and they function to define and protect it. They are the main site of the seven Dhatu Agni as was indicated in earlier lessons. The Kala allow the basic food substance for the tissue to be filtered from the waste products. They are important parts of the Ayurvedic view of anatomy which also should be memorized. They are:

1. SLESHMA DHARA KALA, the membrane that holds Kapha
2. PITTA DHARA KALA, the membrane that holds Pitta
3. MAMSA DHARA KALA, the membrane that holds muscle
4. MEDO DHARA KALA, the membrane that holds fat
5. PURISHA DHARA KALA, the membrane that holds feces
6. MAJJA DHARA KALA, the membrane that holds marrow & nerve
7. SHUKRA DHARA KALA, the membrane that holds reproductive fluid

Most of these are named after their respective Dhatu, like Mamsa dhara kala, the membrane that holds muscle for muscle. The others are named after their respective waste material. The membranes not only serve to feed the tissue but to filter out the waste materials. Therefore, they can be named in either way.

Kapha, also called "Shleshma", is the waste material of Rasa dhatu and Pitta of Rakta dhatu. Pitta dhara kala is also the membrane of the gastro intestinal tract and is responsible for much of the digestive process for the body as a whole.

The membrane for the bones is named after the lining of the colon, as this is its site in the body. Vata is absorbed mainly through the colon and the nutrients to feed the bones are taken in at this place also. The positive side of Vata (Prana) will be absorbed into the bones as the vital energy for the deeper tissues of the body. The treatment of the colon is essential for most Vata and bone disorders as it is the main site of micro-nutrient absorption.

Miscellaneous Concepts in Ayurvedic Anatomy and Physiology

The Divisions of the Body

In Ayurveda Sushruta & Caraka divided the body into six major parts. The Bhavaprakasha gives the following version with eight major parts:

1) Head
2) Neck
3) Arms

4) Chest
5) Abdomen
6) The flanks or sides of the body
7) Back of the body
8) Legs

This is a classic way of describing the body and anatomy in Ayurveda that is still used today. The organs and glands are given their locations according to above divisions of the body. This is interesting but not as useful for the modern application of Ayurveda in a clinical context.

The Marmas

The Marmas, or vital points, of the body are another important part of Ayurvedic anatomy. The Marmas are defined as the junction of the following physical body parts: Veins, Tendons, Joints, Muscle and Bone. There are 107 Marmas and damage to them is considered to cause death or major health problems. They are divided into five kinds:
1) Cause death immediately
2) Cause death after a delay of time
3) Cause deformation of the body
4) Cause chronic pain
5) Cause death when a foreign object is removed (arrow, spear, etc.)

The Marmas are important in diagnosis and treatment of many diseases. The Marmas need to be learned from a teacher and from charts. Most Marmas are simple to understand as they are located at the joints (knee, ankle, etc.) or major organs (heart, navel, etc.).

Marmas are similar to the pressure points used in reflexology and acupressure. Some people believe that the system of Marmas is the origin of reflexology, acupressure and acupuncture. Their use in the context of the Ayurvedic system greatly enhances therapeutic results of any treatment. Like in acupuncture, the Marmas are measured by finger units or *Anguli*. There are 107 magma points and the Astanga Hrdayam further divides them in to six divisions:

"Marma is that place which has unusual throbbing and pain on touch. The Marmas (vital spots) are so called because they cause death; and they are the meeting place of muscle, bones, tendons, arteries, veins, and joints, life entirely resides in them (any injury or assault to these cause danger to life). They are indicated by the predominant structure found in them; on this basis the Marmas are of six kinds. They are one kind only on the common factor, "as seats of life.""

121

The six divisions that Vagbhata refers to are as follows:
1. Mamsa marmas -   are a predominance of muscle tissue
2. Asthi marmas -   have a predominance of bone
3. Snayu marmas -   have a predominance of tendons and ligaments
4. Dhamani marmas -   are a predominance of arteries
5. Sira marmas -   are a predominance of veins
6. Sandhi marmas -   have a predominance of bony joints

The Marmas are further defined by their location and number on the body:
1. Head and Neck-   37
2. Front of the Body -   12
3. Upper Limbs -   22
4. Back of the Body -   14
5. Lower Limbs -   22

Total   107

The majority of information on the Marmas in the ancient texts describes them by the signs they show when they are injured or damaged in some way. Their locations are extremely important to know for accidents, injuries and wounds to the body. As this constitutes the majority of information in the Ayurvedic texts a practitioner who specializes in the treatment of sports injuries, trauma or accidents should research this subject further. The Marma points are mainly areas where Vata Dosha functions. There follows a chart that explains the functional nature of the Marmas in anatomy and physiology. It is helpful to memorize the main Marma points. I personally found that I already knew many of the Marmas because of my previous experience of bodywork. The Marma points need not be seen as a complicated and difficult system, they are naturally sensitive points that may already be known from bodywork.

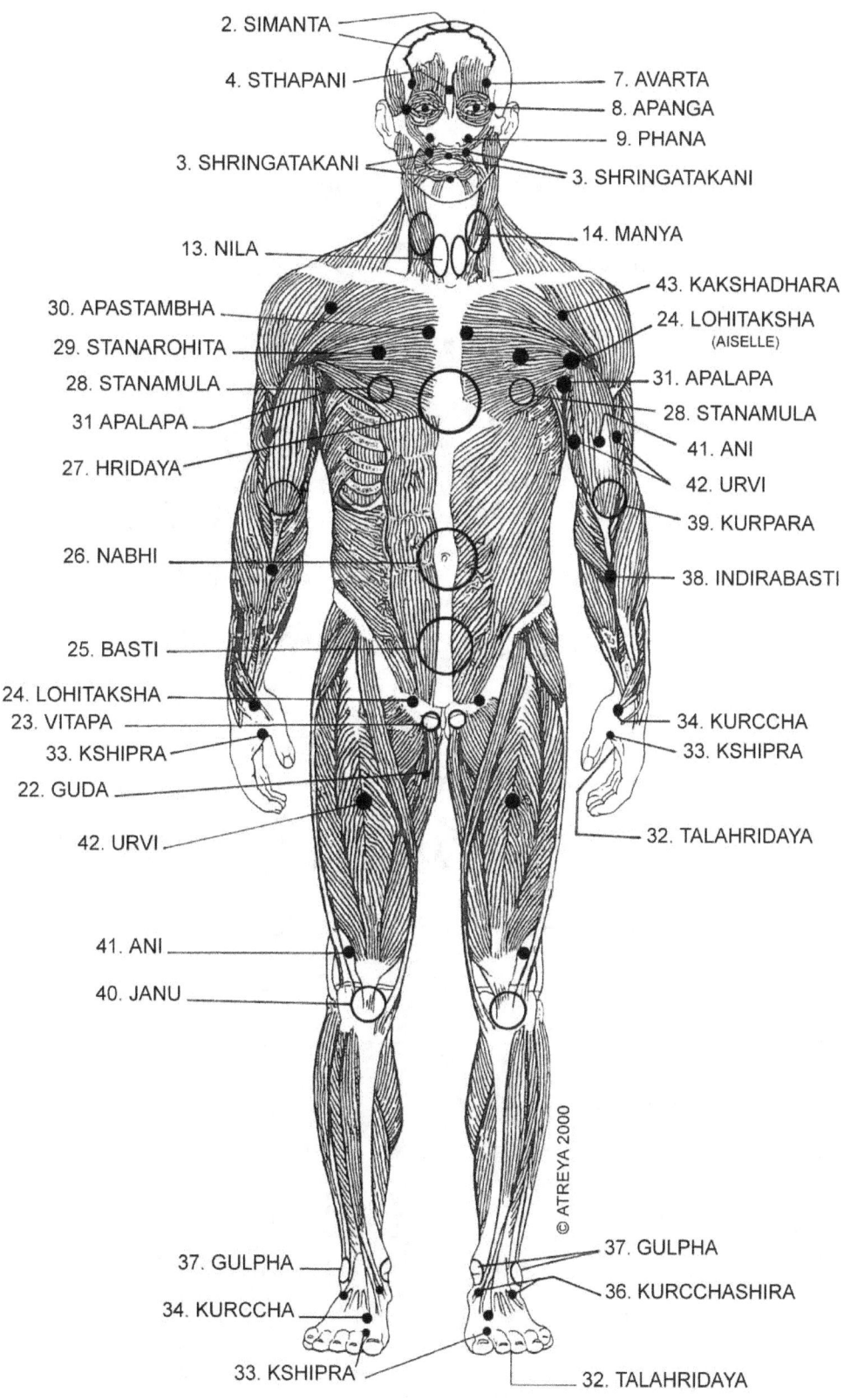

2. SIMANTA

4. STHAPANI

7. AVARTA

8. APANGA

9. PHANA

3. SHRINGATAKANI

3. SHRINGATAKANI

13. NILA

14. MANYA

30. APASTAMBHA

43. KAKSHADHARA

29. STANAROHITA

24. LOHITAKSHA
(AISELLE)

28. STANAMULA

31. APALAPA

31 APALAPA

28. STANAMULA

27. HRIDAYA

41. ANI

42. URVI

39. KURPARA

26. NABHI

38. INDIRABASTI

25. BASTI

24. LOHITAKSHA

23. VITAPA

34. KURCCHA

33. KSHIPRA

33. KSHIPRA

22. GUDA

42. URVI

32. TALAHRIDAYA

41. ANI

40. JANU

37. GULPHA

37. GULPHA

36. KURCCHASHIRA

34. KURCCHA

33. KSHIPRA

32. TALAHRIDAYA

© ATREYA 2000

MARMA POINTS ON THE FRONT OF THE BODY

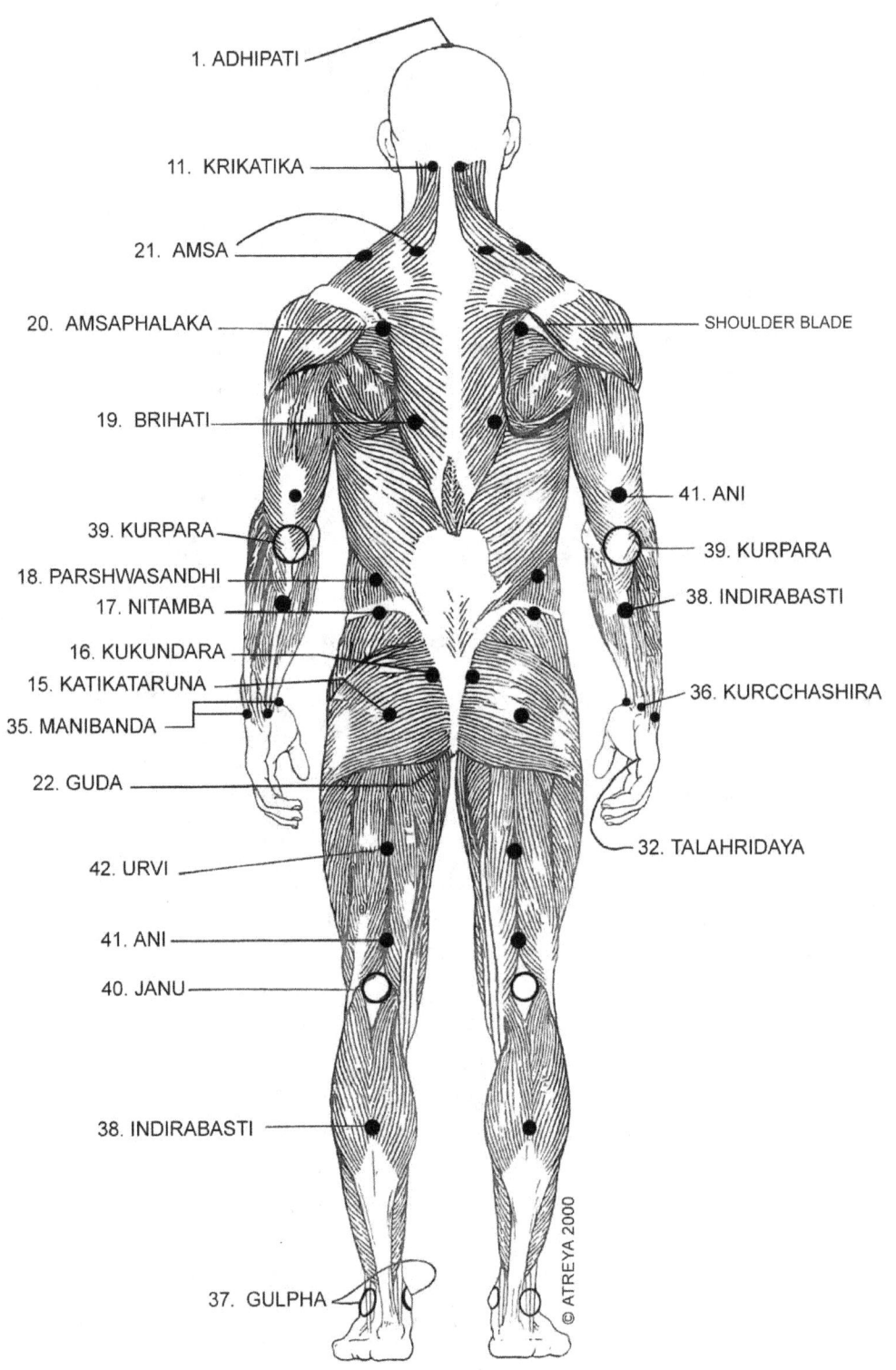

1. ADHIPATI

11. KRIKATIKA

21. AMSA

20. AMSAPHALAKA

SHOULDER BLADE

19. BRIHATI

41. ANI

39. KURPARA

39. KURPARA

18. PARSHWASANDHI

38. INDIRABASTI

17. NITAMBA

16. KUKUNDARA

15. KATIKATARUNA

36. KURCCHASHIRA

35. MANIBANDA

22. GUDA

42. URVI

32. TALAHRIDAYA

41. ANI

40. JANU

38. INDIRABASTI

© ATREYA 2000

37. GULPHA

MARMA POINTS ON THE BACK OF THE BODY

Tables of Marma Points
Head and Neck   *(Please note that sizes are given in anguli, or finger widths.)*

N°	Name & Size	Quantity	Location	Composition	Function
1.	Adhipati 4 anguli	1	top of head	joint in Skull	controls mind, nerves & prana vayu
2.	Simanta goes linear	5	on joints of skull bones	joint in Skull	controls nerves & prana vayu
3.	Shringatakani 1/2 anguli	4	soft palate	blood	controls nerves & prana vayu
4.	Sthapani 1/2 anguli	1	between eyebrows	blood vessels	controls mind, nerves, endocrine glands & prana vayu
5.	Utkshepa 1/2 anguli	2	above Shankha	ligament	controls large intestine & apana vayu
6.	Shankha 2 anguli	2	temple between ear & Apanga	bone	controls large intestine & apana vayu
7.	Avarta 1/2 anguli	2	above eyebrows on the sides	joint	controls vision, alochaka Pitta, & prana vayu
8.	Apanga 1/2 anguli	2	corners of the eyes	blood vessels	controls vision, alochaka Pitta & prana vayu
9.	Phana 1/2 anguli	2	both sides of the nostrils	blood vessels	controls the sinus & prana vayu
10	Vidhura 1/2 anguli	2	below both ears	tendon	controls hearing, balance prana vayu
11	Krikatika 1/2 anguli	2	junction of head & neck	joint	controls neck & shoulder tension & udana vayu
12	Sira Matrika 4 anguli	8	four arteries on each side of the neck	arteries	circulation of the blood to the head and heart, vyana vayu
13	Nila 4 anguli	2	on each side of the larynx	blood vessel	circulation, hoarse voice, udana vayu
14	Manya 4 anguli	2	back of Nila	blood vessel	controls blood circulation, vyana vayu

Back of the Body

N°	Name	Quantity	Location	Composition	Function
15	Katikataruna 1/2 anguli	2	buttocks on center of hip	bone	controls adipose tissue, vyana vayu
16	Kukundara 1/2 anguli	2	next to the sacrum, posterior	joint	controls apana vayu

N°	Name	Quantity	Location	Composition	Function
			superior Iliac spine		
17	Nitamba 1/2 anguli	2	4 anguli above and across from the Kukundara	bone	controls kidneys, apana vayu
18	Parshwasandhi 1/2 anguli	2	2 anguli above Nitamba	blood vessel	controls adrenal & endocrine glands, prana & samana vayu
19	Brihati 1/2 anguli	2	between the 7th & 8th thoracic vertebra	blood vessel	controls samana vayu
20	Amsaphalaka 1/2 anguli	2	on shoulder blades above Brihati	bone	controls prana & vyana vayu
21	Amsa 1/2 anguli	2	4 anguli above Amsaphalaka, between shoulder and neck	ligament	controls udana vayu

Front of the Body

N°	Name	Quantity	Location	Composition	Function
22	Guda 4 anguli	1	around anus	muscular	controls reproductive, urinary, menstrual systems & apana vayu
23	Vitapa 1 anguli	2	2 anguli below Lohitaksha, at the root of the scrotum	muscle and ligaments	controls impotence, fertility, hernia, constipation, menstrual problems & apana vayu
24	Lohitaksha 1/2 anguli	4	joint of groin or shoulders on lymph nodes	blood vessels	controls lymphatic system, circulation & vyana vayu
25	Basti 4 anguli	1	top of pubic bone	ligament	controls Kapha generally & apana vayu
26	Nabhi 4 anguli	1	around navel	ligament	controls small intestine, Pachaka Pitta & samana vayu
27	Hridaya 4 anguli	1	middle of sternum	blood vessel	controls Sadhaka Pitta & Vyana Vayu
28	Stanamula 2 anguli	2	just below the nipples	blood vessels	controls heart, high / low blood pressure, circulation, sadhaka Pitta & vyana vayu

N°	Name	Quantity	Location	Composition	Function
29	Stanarohita 1/2 anguli	2	2 anguli above Stanamula	muscular	controls the breasts, increases milk production, prana & vyana vayu
30	Apastambha 1/2 anguli	2	between the nipples and collar bone	blood vessels	controls the lungs & vyana vayu
31	Apalapa 1/2 anguli	2	lateral side of the Stanamula	blood vessels	controls blood circulation to arms & vyana vayu

Hands and Legs

N°	Name	Quantity	Location	Composition	Function
32	Talahridaya 1/2 anguli	4	in the center of both the palms and the soles	muscular	controls the lungs, heart to some degree & vyana vayu
33	Kshipra 1/2 anguli	4	between the thumb & index finger - and the first and second toes	tendons	controls the heart, prana & vyana vayu
34	Kurccha 1 anguli	4	2 anguli above Kshipra, root of thumb or 1st toe	tendon	foot controls Alochaka Pitta, hand controls prana vayu
35	Kurcchashira 1 anguli	4	Just below wrist joint, or in front of the ankle joint	tendon	controls the stomach, pachaka Pitta & samana vayu
36	Manibanda 2 anguli	2	on wrist joint	joint	controls wrist, stimulates nerves & vyana vayu
37	Gulpha 2 anguli	2	on ankle joint	joint	controls ankles, sciatica, arthritis & vyana vayu
38	Indirabasti 1/2 anguli	4	in the mid-forearm & mid-calf regions	muscular	controls Agni, small intestine, pachaka Pitta & samana vayu
39	Kurpara 3 anguli	2	on elbow	joint	controls liver, spleen & ranjaka Pitta & samana vayu
40	Janu 3 anguli	2	on knee	joint	controls liver, spleen & ranjaka Pitta & samana vayu

41	Ani 1/2 anguli	4	on the arms and legs 3 anguli above Kurpara & Janu	tendon	controls kidneys & apana vayu
42	Urvi 1 anguli	4	in the middle of the upper arm or thigh	blood vessels	controls Amhuvahasrota, vyana & apana vayu
43	Kakshadhara 1 anguli	2	2 anguli above Lohitaksha in shoulder joint	ligament	controls shoulders & vyana vayu

As stated earlier Marmas are measured by finger units, Anguli. This means the width of the finger *of the patient*. Not your own finger. Many of the locations of Marmas are given in this way because each person is made differently and has a different size and proportion. Marmas also differ as compared to other systems in that they vary from one half to four finger widths - often indicating a region of the body and not a point.

The order and numbering of the Marmas in these charts is my own system that I use when teaching this information. I have been teaching the therapeutic use of the Marmas in Ayurvedic bodywork since 1997. The order I use in the charts is reversed somewhat from the tradition; however, I find it works better for way in which I teach Westerners. The correlation to the five vayus is mostly my own. I find this system of naming the Marmas, their locations, and descriptions to be the most accurate. There are other systems, most notably that of South India and Sri Lanka. The South India model has a difference of terminology rather than of its actual nature. The Sri Lanka model may be different due to the strong Buddhist influence, as reflected in many forms of Ayurveda coming from there.

Treatment Methods

The Marmas are primarily treated with pressure, massage and medicated oils. They can also be treated with heat. They are very delicate points on the body and should not be approached forcefully or aggressively. The main concept to understand about the Marmas is that they work on Vata Dosha. Through Vata, Pitta and Kapha can be modified. This is a perfect example of Ayurveda as a functional system of medicine – the Marmas are a methodology in which to use Vata functions to modify Pitta and Kapha functions. Treatments methods of Marmas is covered in Volume Two of this series of textbooks.

The Ten Resorts of Life (Caraka Samhita, Sutrasthana, Ch. 29, Sutra 3)

Ten important sites in the body are recognized in Ayurveda as key to health. These are:
The two temples (2)
The three main vital organs (heart, bladder and head) (3)
The throat (1)
The blood (1)
Reproductive fluid (1)
Ojas (1)
Rectum (1)

Some are sensitive areas, damage to which can cause death, like a blow to the temple, head or chest (heart), breaking the neck or cutting the throat – all of these are Marmas. Others are sensitive tissues, like blood, reproductive fluid or Ojas, loss of which causes de-vitalization of the body and death. Others are important organs whose dysfunction leads to de-vitalization and death, like the head (brain), heart, bladder and rectum. When the bladder does not function properly the tissues become toxic. The same is true to a lesser extent when the colon fails to remove mala from the body.

Problems with these areas in the body can indicate long term problems with vitality. These areas also hold significant amounts of Prana in a vulnerable state and damage to them can hence cause the Prana to be lost or reduced in the body.

Study Questions for Chapter Nine

1. Why are the organs and glands are part of the seven Dhatus in Ayurveda?

2. Which organs and glands is Rasa Dhatu is responsible for the manufacturing and maintenance of?

3. Meda Dhatu is responsible for the manufacturing and maintenance of the kidneys and in a secondary, supporting function to what other organ or gland?

4. Which organs and glands can the Pranavaha Srotas can relate to?

5. Which organs and glands can the Raktavaha Srotas can relate to?

6. Which organs and glands does Vata Dosha primarily relate to?

7. In general how do the three doshas relate to the organs and glands?

8. The heart is a Pitta organ by function and a Kapha organ by structure. Explain why.

9. How do the reproductive organs and glands for men and women relate to the doshas?

10. Which doshas and sub-doshas relates to the hypothalamus?

CHAPTER TEN
INTRODUCTION TO PRAKRITI

This is an introduction chapter to the concept of *Prakriti*. There are four chapters on this subject of how to understand and diagnose Prakriti. There are a number of misconceptions concerning Prakriti – everything from saying that it is not in the classics, to ridged stereotypes, to every possible extreme. One of the main miss-understandings around Prakriti concerns the psychology. These four chapters will try to present the Prakriti concept in a logical, linear manner; all four chapters need to be considered.

We all have one thing in common: we are human beings with three Doshas working together to keep us alive. Yet, according to Ayurveda, we are all unique. We each possess a unique constitution which determines our body-type, metabolic nature and mental orientation. This is called the *constitution*, or as it is called in Ayurveda, the Prakriti, which literally means 'nature'. Caraka uses both *Dehaprakriti* and *Dosaprakriti* to indicate physical constitution. Ayurveda says that your Prakriti is mainly due to the combination of your parents' sperm and ovum, as well as their Dosha predominance at the moment of conception.

"Prakriti or physical constitution of the fetus is determined by the following factors:
- The sperm and ovum.
- The season and condition of the uterus
- The diet and behavior of the mother (before and during pregnancy)
- Nature of the Mahabhutas comprising the fetus

The dosha, one or more, which predominates in these factors, gets attached to the fetus, and is known as "dosaprakriti" (physical or dosika constitution)."
CS.VIM.8.95

This means, among other things, that a person's Prakriti can be independent from the Prakriti of the parents. This happens when either the mother of father are in a state of *Vikriti* (imbalanced doshas) at the time of conception, or during pregnancy (for the mother). Or it can simple mean that the dominate dosha at the time of conception is different than the constitution of the parents. An example of this could be that during conception passion (a Pitta emotion) is dominating. Or one of the parents is worried about something and Vata dominates. It is nice to leave the door open to other possible explanations than Vikriti – which is basically pathology.

Caraka goes on to explain that there are basically seven fundamental Prakriti-types (three pure types, three dual types, and one balanced or tri-doshic type):

"Therefore, some persons are constitutionally slesmala (having predominance of Kapha), some are Pittala and some are vattala, some others have combinations of two dosas and some have equilibrium of three doshas."
CS.VIM.8.95

These three doshas combine to make the seven constitutional types as mentioned above. They are:

1. **Vata** dominant
2. **Pitta** dominant   - Three 'pure' types
3. **Kapha** dominant

4. **Vata-Pitta** dominant
5. **Vata-Kapha** dominant   - Three 'duel' or 'mixed' types
6. **Pitta-Kapha** dominant

7. **Vata-Pitta-Kapha** dominant   - One rarer 'balanced' type.

Ayurveda uses these seven classifications in order to understand the main differences in metabolic types. The question here is not of good or bad, but of biologic differences. By understanding how your metabolism functions you can begin to work with it and not against it. Working against it brings various problems and can eventually lead to diseases of both a minor or severe nature. Working with it brings good digestion and health – not just freedom from disease – but real health.

It is also recognized that there is a huge variance in each type. The main seven types are not to be seen as a final stopping point, but rather as a starting point. We can, once we know our type according to Ayurveda, begin to work in the context of the guidelines for our type. I have experienced this over and over again in my practice.

People will generally already have recognized that certain foods are problematic for them and have learned to avoid them. When they see food recommendations for their type they are amazed to see the foods that are problematic for them should be eliminated according to Ayurveda. However, they often think that these recommendations are final. In reality the recommendations in this course and any book on Ayurvedic nutrition are the basic guidelines which then need to be adjusted and refined to the individual.

The purpose of the seven types, V, P, K, VP, VK, PK and VPK, is not to classify people. It is rather a way to understand how the metabolism functions. In Ayurveda there is never the idea to use one type as a comparison to another type. Actually, it is against the precepts of Ayurveda to compare people in any way shape or form. No constitution is better or worse than any other. Nor, is any one mix or combination better than any other. Each type or combined type has its pros and cons. Actually, everyone has all three principles

– this is just a distinction of which one is dominating the metabolic functions. The dominant dosha indicates the Prakriti.

Occasionally, you will find people using these metabolic distinctions as a means to manipulate, criticize or 'put down' others. Please note that this has nothing to do with the Ayurvedic system. People who feel the need to dominate or criticize others do so from their own insecurity and neurosis – these people will twist any system or means for their own ends. I mention this because it is quite common today for people to judge others and, unfortunately, some people are trying to use Ayurveda in this manner as well. Be clear that there is no value judgment in regard to the different constitutional types.

In order for us to follow the methodology of Ayurveda we need to have a minimal understanding of the seven different types. In general, the seventh type, VPK, is considered quite rare as it indicates an equal amount of the three doshas. This is also my practical experience. I have come across only four types like this in twenty-five years of clinical practice. Therefore, most people will fall under one of the six main types.

To conclude this introduction on the subject of Prakriti, study the overall physical and mental tendencies of the seven Prakriti-types. Once you are familiar with this information, you are ready to learn the protocol that we use in Ayurveda to evaluate someone's Prakriti.

Physical Profiles – An Overview

Vata Prakriti

This person has a variable metabolism; in other words, there is no daily consistency in digestion. One day the person will digest a pizza easily and the next not at all. On still yet another day the same pizza will cause minor indigestion. This shows an inconsistency in metabolism, and as digestive function is one of the main indications of the overall metabolism we can judge that Vata people will not consistently digest the same food or dish the same way.

These people tend to digest quickly when they do digest and tend to get gas when they do not digest well. When this type is disturbed they will become constipated, or bloated, or just 'gassy'. These people will tend to have dry skin, dry hair and it is this same internal dryness that can cause constipation.

This type will generally have a smaller bone structure – their skeletal frame. The bones themselves will be thinner rather than thicker. They will tend to be tall and thin or short and thin. However, when this type is disturbed or agitated they can become fat. This is truer in adulthood after the age of thirty. These people are usually thin by the time they enter adolescence, if not for their whole life.

This type has difficulty to gain weight. No matter how much they eat they rarely seem to gain any weight. In general they are not big eaters, but prefer to eat smaller amounts more frequently. They are the least interested in food of the seven types and will very often settle for poor quality foods like fast foods, junk foods or snacking, just because of a lack of interest.

Even though their metabolism is variable they will tend to be cool or cold most of the time. Their blood circulation is not strong and they generally have cold hands and feet because of this. They do not like cold weather much and need to cover themselves from the elements more than the other types.

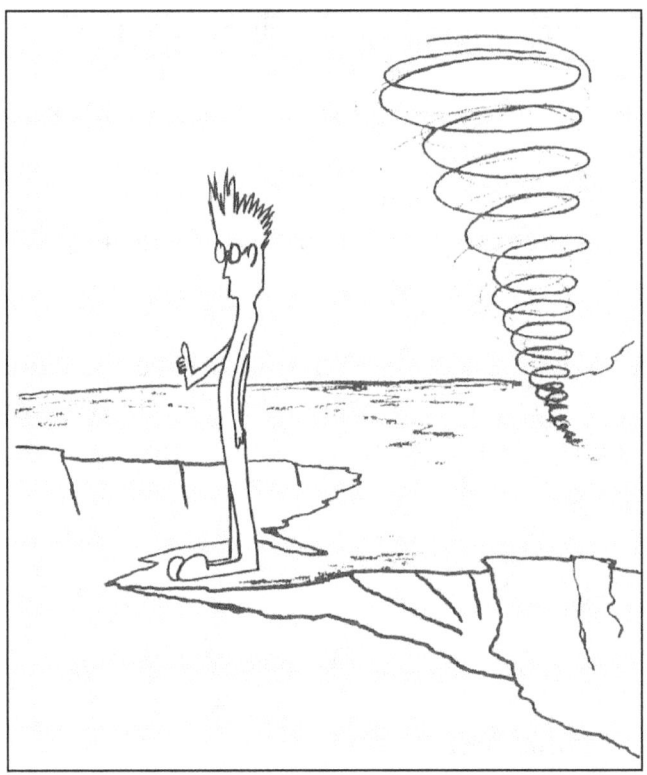

The Vata person has the weakest immune system of all the types and will often come down with allergies, a cold or the flu. Yet, they usually have abundant energy, though not necessarily the stamina to keep up with it. They very often will be quite talkative, or even chaotic in a scattered sort of way. They are known to be good at starting things and not at finishing them. They can easily be disturbed from computers or other electronic devices, as they are the most physically sensitive of the three types.

Pitta Prakriti

The Pitta person has a very strong metabolism. They digest quickly and have the strongest power of digestion; they can eat anything. Their metabolism runs on the hot side and they tend to be 'hot blooded' in all senses of the meaning. They have warm skin, hands and feet. Their blood circulation is the strongest of the three types and they can be prone to heart or blood problems later in life.

Their metabolism is not only strong, but also consistent. Up until about forty years of age they will hardly notice the process of digestion unless it is heart burn or acidity. After forty they begin to notice that a few pounds arrived uninvited. Then they tend to become more aware of problematic foods like tomatoes or acidic citrus fruits.

When they do have problems digestively it reveals itself in the form of loose stools or diarrhea. Fried foods especially can trigger this kind of response. This is extremely true for fast foods or restaurant foods that are prepared in old or poor quality oils. The excess consumption of fried foods can also make them obese. Generally, they are neither thin nor overweight unless they eat too many fried and fatty foods. They will be the most regular in bowel movements of the three types.

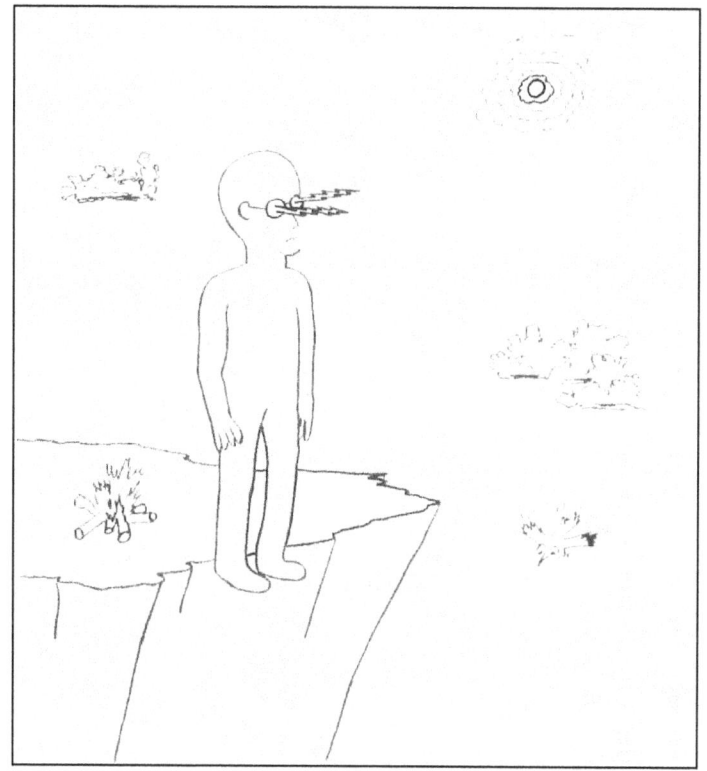

Pitta types tend to suffer from skin problems due to the acidic nature of their blood and body fluids in general. They can also have liver problems even if they do not drink alcohol. Their eyesight may be poor or they may have trouble with their eyes at some point in their life. Generally, they will tend to have red eyes or be sensitive to the sunlight more than the other types. They often wear glasses.

They tend to be medium in build and bone structure. They are the most 'average' in size of the three types. However, do not be deceived by this distinction. Any of the types can have an 'average' build. They fall in-between the other types in both size and weight. They have an average level of endurance and stamina. Nonetheless, they have the strongest minds and so they can achieve actions beyond their normal strength or stamina through will power alone.

They have a good immune system and do not generally fall sick – unless they work too much! They tend to suffer more from frustration or over work than from physical illness.

They are prone to exhaustion and burn out which leaves them open to infectious diseases. They usually suffer from inflammatory problems when they do fall ill.

Kapha Prakriti

This person has the slowest metabolism, but the greatest consistency. Their digestive capacity is very regular and consistent. They can easily become congested or overloaded as their metabolism functions slowly. Of the three types these people take the longest to process what they eat. They will respond regularly to the same kinds of foods or meals.

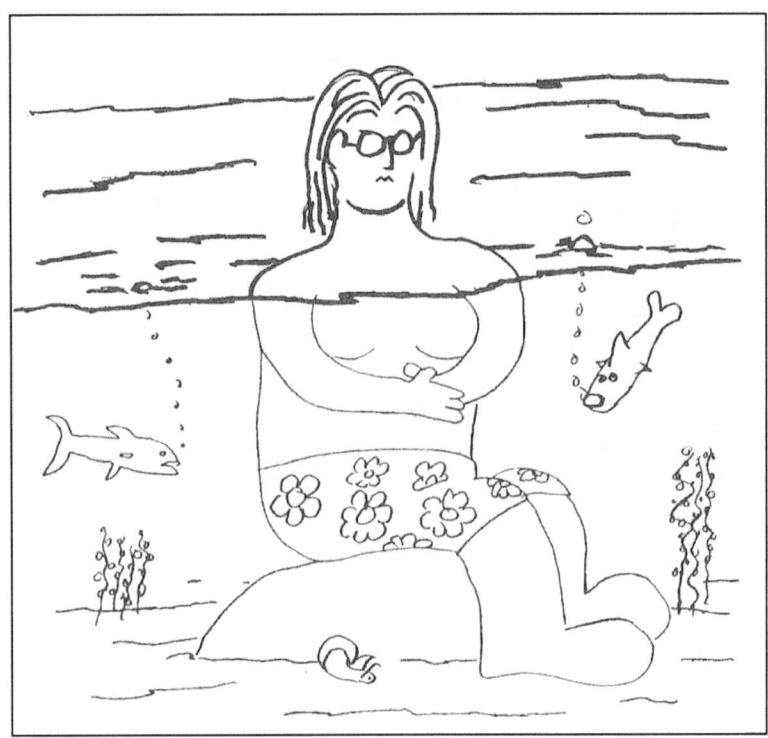

When they have digestive disturbances they will get bloated or have a subjectively heavy feeling in the stomach or abdomen area. As their digestion reflects their slow metabolic function they can easily over eat or eat too much of heavy, slow to digest foods. Disturbances tend to be reflected in accumulation of mucus or fat as when the intake of food is greater than the metabolic ability of processing and assimilation.

These people have the least resistance to sweets. Yet, they may be the most attracted to eating them of all the types. This attraction can put an extra strain on the adrenal – pancreas function that regulates blood sugar and the processing of fats and cholesterol among other things. Their kidney function can also become weak from any excess fat that is accumulated. Of the three types they will hold more weight in fluids because of the inherent weakness in the water metabolism – i.e., kidney function. This can give a 'puffy' look to the skin and edema in general.

Kapha people have the strongest body and the greatest level of endurance of the three types. While somewhat prone to becoming over weight, it is by no means mandatory. They can achieve great feats of strength in certain sports and types of professions. They are the most physically orientated of the types and so have the greatest attraction for food. They have the largest bone structure of the three types yet tend to be strong, of medium height, and stocky.

Along with their physical strength they have the strongest immune function. Their resistance to disease is much greater than the other types and Kapha people will generally not become sick. When they do become ill it usually reflects poor nutritional or lifestyle habits. This includes drinking alcohol and smoking both of which cause problems for all the types. The Kapha type is prone to all kinds of accumulation in the body. This can manifest as tumors and other internal growths – of a benign nature. They can also be prone to lung problems or problems of the respiratory system in general.

The Kapha type generally enjoys the greatest level of physical health. Provided they do not indulge in extremes these people can live the longest and healthiest of the types. However, if they indulge in poor habits and nutrition they can fall ill and die from the many diseases of an affluent society.

Vata/Pitta Prakriti

This type is a mix of both Vata and Pitta. These mixes are called dual types as they reflect a combination of both principles. Usually, a dual type is pretty equal in displaying the traits of their type. However, one of the types can dominate in either the body or the psychology giving a person who looks like one type but behaves like another type. This is not the typical scenario, however, and is an exception to the rule.

Physically these types are in-between the Vata and Pitta types or following either the Vata or the Pitta type. Generally, they are thinner rather than thicker and can exhibit either the dry, nervous qualities of the Vata type or the hot, dynamic qualities of the Pitta type. As nature is infinite in her combinations so are the possible mixes of these two principles. Physical structure is less a means of determining a dual type than observing your metabolism. This kind of mix will tend to have a strong digestion but be occasionally troubled by gas, malabsorption of nutrients, or diarrhea. They will normally be free from disease and are stronger than the pure Vata type. Yet, they are not as resistant to illness as the Pitta type and can – when unbalanced – fall prey to the problems of both Vata and Pitta.

On the same tract, this mix can also exhibit the best attributes of the two types. This combination can make good athletes like track and field, skiing, racing or any sort, or swimming. They like to move and compete in events or activities and are perhaps more social than the pure Pitta type. They are also easier going than the pure Pitta type, yet more practical and persistent than the pure Vata type.

As the Vata person is the most innovative and creative and the Pitta person is the most practical and dynamic, this type is revered in our present society. The more developed side of this mix is a person who can achieve many things that are creative and innovative. They communicate well and are full of energy. They have the ability to actualize their ideas and dreams in concrete forms and can make good leaders in business. This is also an excellent mix for teaching in general and the pursuit of knowledge. The Pitta qualities add a good determination to the Vata qualities for the pursuit of studies and the ability to focus on one subject at a time in order to fully explore it.

In less developed types this mix can lead to intellectual indecisiveness, insecurity and frustration. They can become over mental but with a frustration or sense of irritability that can be difficult to live with. This mix can also lead to irrational kinds of behavior with a violent or aggressive flavor if the mind is disturbed.

Vata/Kapha Prakriti

The Vata/Kapha mix is an interesting mixture that can offer great qualities or conflicts. The physical nature of this type will tend to reflect the Kapha type more than the Vata type of body; i.e., stronger and well-formed rather than thin. In a smaller percentage of people the Vata type can dominate physically, but if this is the case, the mental disposition will exhibit more Kapha type qualities.

Physically this type can suffer from some of the traits of the Vata type like dry constipation and colic pain. Generally speaking, this type has a strong constitution and does not become ill very easily. They do, however, tend to be troubled by many small, nagging problems in their health. These problems are usually related to the Vata principle and reflect either migrating pains, nervous problems or irregularities in the metabolism. The Vata side of the constitution can aggravate the Vata side quite effortlessly and cause bloating, distension, and edema. The lungs can also suffer from allergies or congestion. The Kapha side can cause congestive problems like constipation, edema or weight gain.

The easiest qualities of this combination are the intuitive, quick mental attributes of the Vata type together with the stability and persistence of the Kapha type. The farsighted Kapha type counteracts the usual short sightedness of the Vata type – this combination gives many qualities for artistic endeavors. This type can be very socially oriented and can work well with people in a caring, motherly capacity. They make good service oriented people and are good at communicating and relating with others.

When afflicted they can suffer from the worst of both principles. This can be hard to deal with, as qualitatively the two are opposites. This means that the Vata side likes to move and change while the Kapha side hates change and movement. The Vata type likes all kinds of irregularity – staying up late, eating at strange hours – and the Kapha type likes regularity – eating and sleeping at the same time every day. The physical problems that can result from this are reflected in a confused metabolism.

The slowness of the Kapha side is quite disturbed by the erratic behavior of the Vata side. The spontaneity of the Vata side is aggravated by the rigidity of the Kapha side. Understanding the two sides is critical for this combination or mental and physical unhappiness results. Working with the dual aspect of the constitution brings harmony and peaceful metabolic function. Ignoring one or the other of these sides will bring digestive, nervous disorders and mental problems – usually poor self-esteem and self-negating attitudes. This can be one of the most interesting and happy of the types when both sides of the nature are well understood.

Pitta/Kapha Prakriti

This type is very good for competitive sports and physically demanding activities. The strong will of the Pitta type combines with the strong body of the Kapha type and gives a powerful combination. Most of our sports heroes in football and basketball are of this type. The mental discipline needed to routinely exercise and practice is a quality of the Kapha type and the competitive, fighting quality reflects the Pitta type.

These types physically are quite strong – the strongest in many ways – as they not as prone to become congested by the accumulation of the Kapha principle. Their metabolism runs hotter and stronger than the Kapha type, yet not too hot or acidic as the pure Pitta type. This is a good combination for physical activities. The problem can be if the people become sedimentary and stagnant in the life. This will tend to aggravate both sides of the constitution. The Pitta side will become congested by the Kapha qualities as they increase in dominance. The more inactive this type is the more problems they will have.

Mentally this type needs challenge or they become unhappy and discontented. However, they are not risk takers generally, but rather they plan. The Kapha type is conscious and careful, combined with the Pitta type the person can act when needed – though rarely without planning. These people prefer to work or be active in defined areas, such as their home town or neighborhood. They may travel some or go to the same place for vacation regularly. They are more habitual than the other mixed types.

This type can also make a CEO executive type of person. While the Kapha type is good with people and management the Pitta type is aggressive and seeks power. To run a business the two qualities are often needed or the person may not be motivated enough, strong enough, or not be able to work well with subordinates sufficiently. Their willingness to fight over long periods of time for a goal gives them a powerful presence even if their physical body is not developed.

These two principles tend to work well together. The physical problems that can arrive are heart problems – especially congestion of the arteries and blood vessels. They are also prone to problems of the pancreas and the gall bladder – both tend to become congested or blocked from poor nutrition and eating habits. These people do have strong appetites so it is important that they eat foods that they are capable of completely digesting. They are prone to eat overly rich and fried foods that – while young – they may be able to digest easily. Although, once in the mid-thirties they can balloon out with sudden weight gain.

Vata/Pitta/Kapha Prakriti

This person has a balanced physical and mental disposition. Traditionally these people are the least likely to become ill or disturbed. If they do become ill it can be from any of the three principles. In our modern culture Vata is the most likely to become unbalanced and disturb the other aspects of the constitution. This is also a traditional understanding of Ayurveda. The Vata is the most irregular and unstable by its nature of movement. As our society loves movement and is less and less attracted to tradition and regularity this increases the tendency even more.

This type of person will tend to have a Pitta/Kapha type of body, stronger rather than thinner. Although thinness is attractive in our culture of top models and our worship of adolescent youth, it is not always conducive to good health. The body needs some fat and good muscle tone. Hence, the equal type, VPK, reflects a stronger frame and tissue make-up than most of the other types. This person is said to be free of disease and unhappiness. They are said to live long and enjoy life. They are also said to be the rarest. Once again it is good to remember that one type is not better than another. *Any of the types can be thrown into a state of unbalance by bad habits and poor nutrition, even the equal type.* Generally, this type will have the greatest capacity to withstand disease and bad habits provided they are temporary and not part of lifetime habits.

This is due to the equilibrium that is present in the combination of the three together. It is the combination of the three that gives strength and freedom from disease, not because one is better than another is or stronger.

Prakriti according to Ashthanga Hridayam

It can be interesting to read how a classic ayurvedic text defines Prakriti. It is interesting to see how they generally favor the Kapha body type over Vata and Pitta. This is mainly for climatic and cultural reasons. Also the Vata type was not good for the family (tribe) continuity as Vata Prakriti people tended to travel and be less interested in the stability of the family. It is important to remember that each body type has its pros and cons and that the Vata / Pitta type we favor today could be culturally negative in a hundred years.

Vata Prakriti according to Ashthanga Hridayam

"Because of (properties like) all pervading (in all the parts of the body), quick acting, strong (powerful), tendency to aggravate others (doshas, dhatus and malas etc.), acting independently, and producing many diseases Vata is powerful among the doshas. Hence persons born with the predominance of pavana (Vata) generally have, hair and body which are cracked and dusky (lusterless), they hate cold, are unsteady in respect of courage, memory, thinking, movement (walking and others), friendship, vision and gait; talk more and irrelevant, possess little of wealth, strength, span of life and sleep; their voice (speaking) is obstructed, interrupted, unsteady or harsh; they are atheists, gluttons, pleasure seeking; desirous of music, humor, hunting or gambling; desirous of habituation to sweet, sour, salty and hot foods; are lean and tall in shape, produce sound during walking (knuckles in joints of the leg); are not steadfast, cannot control their senses, not, civilized (brutish, impolite), not liked by women, not have many children; their eyes are rough (dry), lusterless, round, unpleasant and resemble those of the dead; lids kept open while sleeping; they dream as though roaming on the mountains, dwelling on trees and moving in the sky; persons of Vata Prakriti are non-magnanimous, bloated with jealousy, of stealing nature and having bulged calves; they resemble (in movements, mental behavior etc.) animals such as the dog, jackal, camel, vulture, rat and crow."

Pitta Prakriti according to Ashthanga Hridayam

"Pitta is fire itself or born from fire; hence persons having predominance of Pitta, have very keen (severe) thirst and hunger; are white (in the color of the skin) and warm in body; possess coppery red palms, soles and face; are brave and proud; have brown and scanty hair; are fond of women, garlands, unguents (perfumeries); are of good behavior, clean, affectionate to dependents, desirous of grandeur, adventure have mental power (ability) of facing fear and enmity; highly intelligent, possess very loose and lean joints and muscles; do not like women; possess less of semen and sexual desire; possess grey hair, wrinkles, and blue patches on the skin; consume food which is sweet, astringent, bitter and cold; hate sunlight (and heat); perspire heavily, emit bad smell from the body; expel feces frequently, have more anger, eating, drinking (wine) and jealousy; while in sleep dream of (flowers of) karnikara and palaśa, forest fire, meteor, lightening/thunder bolt, bright sunrays and fire; their eyes are thin (small), brown, unsteady with thin and few eyelashes; eyes desirous of cold comfort, becoming red very quick by anger, drinking wine and exposure to sunlight. Persons of Pitta Prakriti are of medium life-span, medium strength, highly learned, afraid of discomfort and resemble (in behavior) animals like the tiger, bear, ape, cat and yakśa."

Kapha Prakriti according to Ashthanga Hridayam

"Shleshman (Kapha) is soma (moon-like, cool, mild); hence persons of Kapha Prakriti are mild in nature, possess deep seated (not prominently seen), unctuous and well-knit joints and muscles; are not much troubled by hunger, thirst, unhappiness (troubles) strain and heat; endowed with intelligence, right attitude and truthfulness; possess color like that of priyangu, dūrva, śarakanda, śastra (iron, steel weapon), gorocana, padma or suvarna; have long arms, big and elevated chest, big (wide) forehead, thick and blue hair; soft, even (symmetrical), well defined and good looking body, of great vigour, sexual prowess, desire in tastes; more of semen, children and attendants; are of righteous, benevolent nature, do not speak harsh and abusively; harbor enmity, concealed and deep for long time; their gait is like that of an elephant in rut; their voice like the roaring of clouds, ocean, mridanga, (drum) or lion; possess good memory, perseverance, humbleness, do not weep (cry) much even in childhood; are not greedy (clinging to pleasures) consume food which is bitter, astringent, pungent, hot, dry and less in quantity, and still remain strong; their eyes are red at the angles, unctuous, wide, long, with well-defined white and black spheres (sclera and cornea) and with more eye lashes; have less of speech, anger, desire for drink (wine), food and activities; endowed with more life (longevity), wealth, foresight and munificence (generosity); have faith (in god, granting gifts, charity etc.); dignified, greatly charitable; of forgiving nature, civilized; very sleepy/drowsy, slow, grateful, straightforward, learned, pleasant to look at, bashful, obedient, teachers (and elders) and of fast friendship; see reservoirs of water full of lotus and rows of birds and clouds (in dream); persons of shleshman Prakriti are similar (in nature) with Brahma, Rudra, lindra, Varuna, Tarkshya (garuda) hamsa (swan) Gajadhipa (the elephant Airavata), lion, horse, and bull."

Mixed types according to Ashthanga Hridayam

"Persons born with predominance of two doshas and all three doshas possess features of two or all the doshas together."

"Among the seven kinds of dosha Prakriti, persons of sammisra Prakriti (combination of all the three dosha in equal proportion) are the best in health and other aspects but very few in numbers. Persons of samsarga Prakriti (combination of any two dosha) are moderate (in health etc.) and form highest percentage numerically; persons of ekadoshoja Prakriti (single dosha origin) are poor in health and other aspects. Among these three, Kapha Prakriti is best, Pitta Prakriti moderate and Vata Prakriti is least."

Psychological Profiles – An Overview

The physiological function of the three doshas provides the structure and form for the psychology to function – in other words the body – the psychology cannot exist without a body in which it is contained. Therefore, the physical Prakriti of the body tends to influence the mental Prakriti as well – even though the mind is functional in nature it still needs a location, or structure, in which it can function. One can view this as the mind resting in a bowl, which represents the physical structure and is created by the three doshas and seven dhatus. There is a transfer of the physical attributes (twenty Gunas) of the body to the psychology through this structure.

To look at the body without the mind, or to look at the mind without the body, is an error. Logically neither the mind nor the body can exist alone. In fact, the human being is only one entity, it is not two or three (e.g.; mind / body or soul / mind / body). It is simply the nature of the human mind to separate anything in order to better understand it. This is due to the Samkhya principle of Ahamkara which separates and divides. In and of itself this is not a problem; the problem arises because the mind fails to "reassemble" that which it wrongly took apart to understand. Hence, the human being is one being. It is impossible to separate the soul, mind or the body from each other. Therefore, it is logical to assume that there is some influence from the twenty Gunas of the body to the three Maha Gunas that control the functional nature of the mind. While it is not correct to view the mind wholly from the three Doshas it is also not correct to view the mind wholly from the three Gunas ether. The following text try's to illustrate the "structural" aspect of the Prakriti psychology.

This diagram illustrates this idea:

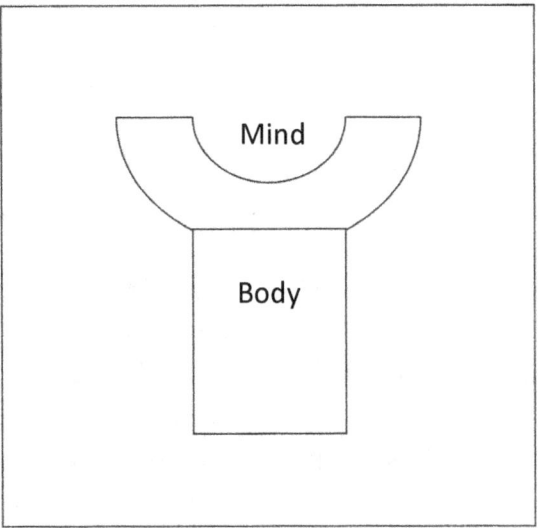

Psychological Profile of Vata Prakriti

The Vata person can be very creative, imaginative and innovative. The Vata type is very good in all forms of abstract thinking or creativity. But they can have problems with the practical side of life. The 'absent minded professor' is a typical Vata type with a scientific bend. They make good artists in all fields of creativity. They are very good in communication and generally like to talk or work in fields of communications.

They are the most spontaneous and flexible of all the types. This is one of their qualities. They like travel and change. In fact, they thrive on change and will change things just for the sake of change – even when it may be quite impractical to do so. They can be very intuitive.

These types are often brilliant intellectually with very quick minds. Yet, their memory is generally not that strong. They are more concerned with the short term and not very interested in the long term. They are the non-conformists of the three types. They may exist on the edges of society, even though they can be very social and likeable. They make poor leaders and even poorer followers. They may be a socialite and enjoy being in society though in a more superficial way with few real friends.

When this type becomes disturbed or unbalanced they suffer from worry, anxiety, nervous tension, nervous breakdowns, fear, and depression. They are the most sensitive of all the types and so suffer more from stress or nervous system problems. These types are the most prone to become perverse or distorted. They can also become addicts easier than the other types. Addiction can affect all types but is common in the Vata type as they are the most sensitive and can easily fall under emotional or physical dominance - by a person or substance.

Psychological Profile of Pitta Prakriti

The Pitta type is the most purposeful and goal oriented of the types. They rarely do anything without a purpose. Even relaxation or sports will have a goal attached to it in some manner. While understanding and focusing on goals is important in life these types tend to become obsessed with the process.

Generally, their motivation is not towards money, but rather power and control. A more developed Pitta type is orientated towards understanding things and knowledge. They are the most motivated of the types. If they are unable to follow a goal or purpose in life they become frustrated or unhappy. They need to have hobbies and interests outside of their profession or they risk to become consumed by their work.

As the Pitta principle in nature controls the transformation of matter these types are good at initiating events. They make good entrepreneurs and generally like positions of responsibility. In any situation these types will gravitate towards the responsible or authoritative positions. They are seldom satisfied to follow or serve unless they respect the person or system in which they work.

When disturbed they can become aggressive and controlling. They usually become frustrated over events that can turn into anger, irritability or jealousy. They have 'hot' emotions and have little difficulty in expressing how they feel. Yet, it is often not done in a manner that is constructive. Rather they tend to explode and then have to put things back together afterwards.

They sometimes surround themselves with less intelligent or more subservient people in order to control others and expand their ego. In the more developed Pitta types this same quality becomes helpful and humanitarian. A developed Pitta person makes a good teacher, leader and helper. They often are found in humanitarian service orientated roles such as social workers, relief workers and the medical profession. Still other Pitta types will become engrossed in the pursuit of knowledge and understanding. In this sense they can become good psychiatrists or psychotherapists.

Psychological Profile of Kapha Prakriti

Psychologically these people are concerned with comfort and security. This interest tends to reflect itself in every sphere of life. In a positive sense it makes a Kapha type caring and wanting to feed and provide for those around them. In a negative sense it turns a person into a controlling, greedy type who is unwilling to share a crust of bread with someone else unless they pay for it.

These two extremes reflect the basic need or desire for security. Emotionally, love is also a form of security. Hence, these people can become obsessed with the need to be loved. This can take on a very sentimental, romantic flare, or a neurotic, needy quality. Remember that everyone has all three types to some extent and each of us has moments when romance is dominating our psychology. The Kapha type is the most concerned by love relationships and by love in general. It can happen through social or family conditioning that this takes on a neurotic flavor, but simply reflects the lower or negative side of this type.

One common tendency with the Kapha type is to replace love with food. When a loving relationship is absent then food becomes disproportionally important to a Kapha type. Food is also a symbolic form of love and it is a very concrete form of security. It can happen that people who feel inferior or unloved will put on large amounts of weight to give themselves more presence around others. These types can also over eat out of a sense of need, which reflects greed for security in the form of food. As their metabolism is the least able to handle excessive amounts of food they often become fat through this psychological tendency.

They are strong and consistent in their efforts, goals and relationships and make a good mate or employee. They tend to like and be close to the people in their family and close friends. They are not very open to change in any way and take time to warm to others outside of their immediate group or friends and family. Yet, they often have the deepest relationships of the three types.

Mentally they are a little slower than the other types – not less intelligent – but slower. They like to reflect over things and think about them before coming to a conclusion about anything. They do not make rash decisions, nor can you push them. Generally, the more you try to push a Kapha person the less he/she will move. They are best communicated with through love and understanding. It can be necessary to be firm and even forceful with Kapha types in order to get them to change bad habits or to help them change. Even this must be done with love or care as they can be very resistant and stubborn.

Mixed psychological profiles show a mixture of traits, or alternate between the two.

Summary of Prakriti or Constitution

Classical Ayurveda points out is that no matter what your constitutional type is men will tend to have more Pitta traits and women will tend to have more Kapha traits. This is a generality that shows the more feminine, caring and receptive side of nature or the Kapha type for women. Men tend to be more aggressive and goal orientated, which reflects the dynamic aspect or nature of the Pitta type.

During the course of the day it is normal for everyone to move through the different types emotionally. Each type reflects certain aspects of human nature; hence, we will tend to have them all at some point in the day or week. What we are trying to establish is which of them is dominant in your nature.

An example could be that during the day I get my children ready for school – feed them, cloth them and help them to on the bus. All of which are Kapha types of emotions and actions. Then I go to work to sell shoes and move into my Pitta emotions and actions. Perhaps I have an inspiration on how to sell more shoes, which reflects the creative side of the Vata psychology. Then I again come home to my spouse and feel romantic, or passionate, Kapha and Pitta types of emotions. And just before sleeping I have an inspiration on how to redecorate the living room, a Vata type of inspiration. Thus, all three doshas manifest themselves psychologically in the day.

Also remember that any one of the types can be positive or negative depending on you. It is up to you if you want to reflect the higher or lower qualities of any constitutional type. This is not fixed genetically. If you want to be a criminal or a humanitarian it is up to you. By the same token, if you want to eat well or eat junk food it is also up to you. Whatever your constitution is you still have the ability to shape and control your life – only now you will be able to work with your nature – whatever it is – and not fight against it.

"Some people maintain the equilibrium of Vata, Pitta and Kapha from conception; some are dominated by Vata, some by Pitta and others by Kapha."
CS.SU.7.39

Study Questions Chapter Ten

1. What is Prakriti determined by?

2. How many types of Prakriti do the classics define?

3. What is main purpose to determine Prakriti?

4. What Prakriti tends to produce Manda Agni (low Agni)?

5. Which Prakriti type tend to find it hard to gain weight?

6. Define Prakriti.

7. Why are certain Prakriti types are better than others?

8. If you have Vata-Pitta Prakriti how will your metabolism function?

9. If you have Pitta-Kapha Prakriti how will your metabolism function?

10. If you have Vata-Kapha Prakriti how will your metabolism function?

CHAPTER ELEVEN
PRAKRITI PARIKSHA - DIAGNOSING PRAKRITI

One of the most misunderstood concepts in Ayurveda is that a practitioner should determine the Prakriti of the patient immediately. Ayurvedic diagnosis is primarily concerned with the function of the three doshas. Thus all diagnostic methods view either the balance or disturbance of the body in terms of excess of the three doshas. Therefore, each person is seen as an individual, not as an average statistic. Aside from this individualized approach the practical reality is that the dosha increase and "cover up" each other, often making the task of determining Prakriti difficult or impossible.

Note that there are two types of diagnose in Ayurvedic medicine:
* Determining the constitution or birth type of the person (*Prakriti pariksha*)
* Determining the imbalance or disease of the person (*Vikriti pariksha*)

Each of these represents a different approach in Ayurveda. The first is concerned with the lifetime constitution or Prakriti. The second corresponds to any temporary, imbalanced state or disease that may pass over the natal constitution. This is called the *Vikriti* in Ayurveda – literally that which "covers the Prakriti". This can be as simple as fatigue, a common cold or a serious disorder such as cancer. The subject of Vikriti will be studied after pathology in Volume Two of this textbook series. Prakriti is part of the normal function of the body and is part of Anatomy and Physiology because it controls both directly.

Remember the quote from Caraka in the last chapter:
"The dosha, one or more, which *predominates* in these factors, gets attached to the fetus, and is known as dosaprakriti (physical or dosika constitution)."
CS.VIM.8.95

Caraka clearly uses the word "predominates" when speaking of Prakriti. When starting *Prakriti Pariksha* it is important to keep in mind that all three doshas are in the body and each is carrying out their role of physiology to make the body function. Thus, the practitioner can "find" all three doshas in every person they try to diagnose. Hence, the key to avoid confusion when determining Prakriti is to look for the "dominate" dosha, knowing full well that the other doshas will be present and carrying out their proper role in the physiology.

This is main reason why traditional Ayurveda studies Anatomy and Physiology before the study of Prakriti. When following this process the student is not confused by the concept of Prakriti because it is simply a reflection of the functional aspects of the metabolism or physiology.

How to Avoid Misdiagnosing Prakriti

Though the basic rules of determining Prakriti apply to everyone, so too do all three dosha exist in every human body. This often makes it difficult to determine which dosha is dominating the metabolism during the lifetime. In order to avoid misdiagnosis we need to be aware of some basic bias that will influence our observations. These common bias are listed below.

Prakriti bias

This is the risk of seeing what we, the practitioner, are familiar with in ourselves and failing to see what is unique in the patient. For example, if the practitioner is a Pitta type, they will tend to see more Pitta attributes in the patient. Be alert of this tendency will lessen the tendency to project the observers natal Prakriti onto the patient being observed. It is not uncommon for new practitioners to diagnose most of their early patients into the same Prakriti as themselves. It is a good idea to re-read the 100 case-studies of clients to see if there is a pattern that emerges.

Another aspect of the Prakriti bias is related to the community the person lives in. For example, if the person has started their ayurvedic practice near an asthanga yoga community, they may attract a crowd of Vata or Pitta type people, and less Kapha type people (Kapha types tend to steer clear of dynamic yoga practices). Or, they may get references from several clients that lead to having a large number of patients from one profession that attracts a certain typology; this is what happened to me in Paris in the mid 1990's when the majority of my patients worked in the fashion industry.

It is my clinical experience that roughly 60% of the population is of mixed or dual types, and the other 40% are pure types. The classical texts indicate that pure types are less common than mixed types. My experience over the twenty-five years supports this point of view.

The Prakriti bias can also represent cultural preferences. In India Kapha types are more valued. In the United States Pitta/Vata types are more valued. In the fashion industry Vata types are valued, etc. This should be taken into account as whatever the cultural conditioning is it will affect the judgment on the Prakriti of others people.

Race bias

Morphology, skin color and hair type vary between races. African people have dark skin and large, full lips. Japanese people have rounder features and pale skin. This can mean that an error in determining Prakriti comes about when working with people from different races if we are not careful. Avoiding race bias error requires that we become familiar, to some extent, with the nuances of each race that we work with. This is a practical concern in the modern world where interracial marriages are common.

Sex bias

Men tend to have a slightly stronger appetite than women and are often slightly hotter metabolism in general. Psychologically, men tend to be more 'fiery' whereas women are more 'watery'. This means that men tend to demonstrate slightly more Pitta dosha traits compared to women, who express slightly more Kapha dosha traits. This is a generalization, but it is important not to compare two people of opposite sex when trying to determine their Prakriti.

Age bias

Another factor to bear in mind when determining Prakriti is age. The doshas are modified with age and follow a logic that is explained later the lessons on pathology. Simplified, it means that children express relatively more Kapha dosha; adults more Pitta dosha, and elderly people more Vata dosha. Care has to be taken to factor this in. Again – the solution to avoiding age bias is to get to know what is normal for each age group.

Genetic bias

A Genetic bias reflects the genetic background of the individual. Some authors write that Vata people are either quite tall or short, and that Pitta people are medium height, and that Kapha people are medium to short. This point of view can hold true, however, it is not always that reliable. Height tends to follow the genetics, meaning that if the patient comes from a line of tall parents, they are more likely to be a tall person *irrespective of their Prakriti*. So when assessing the physical attributes of a person – such as the length of their nose – try to do so *relative to the individual* as opposed to making an empirical measurement compared to the average for all people. When it comes to observing structure and form, this is an important concept; we are looking for the proportions and shape (length versus height) rather than the empirical measure. For example, rather than measuring the length of the fingers and saying "these are long because they are X centimeter's long"; it can be better to say "these fingers are long because compared to their thickness, they are proportional long".

Advise on How to Diagnose

The real problem of diagnosis is that it is 100% subjective. This means that the practitioner who is diagnosing the patient is not objective; they cannot be. The reason why is that the practitioner needs to use their senses to do carry out the diagnosis procedures. The senses receive information and process it with the conditioned min (*Manas*) and the intellect (*Buddhi*). This creates another bias, the bias of subjectivity, that is impossible to avoid, but is possible to minimize. Therefore, it is extremely important that we learn how to reduce this manner in which we collect and process information or knowledge.

Caraka has the following to say about the subject of diagnosis and the acquisition of knowledge in general:

"Everything can be divided into two categories, true or untrue. These can be examined by taking recourse to one of the following four methods:
1) Authoritative statement from a Sage (*Rishi*),
2) Direct perception,
3) Inference,
4) Reasoning."
CS.SU.11.17

This is an important concept to grasp before starting Prakriti diagnosis. Caraka teaches us to understand how we attain knowledge and how to judge the value of that knowledge, thus, reducing subjectivity and increasing objectivity. When this is done the diagnosis is closer to the reality of the patient and less influenced by the psychology of the practitioner.

Definition of the authority of a Sage:

"Those enlightened persons who are absolutely free from the predominance of Rajas and Tamas (i.e., have a pure mind of Sattva) by the virtue of the power of penance have attained uninterrupted knowledge of Past, Present and Future are known as *Aptas*."
CS.SU.11.18

The classic texts in Ayurveda – Caraka Samhita and Susruta Samhita – are the transmissions of Sages or Rishis to their students. This is considered to be the highest form of knowledge in Ayurveda. When a living Rishi is available then it is best to receive knowledge directly from them. When this is not possible then the text, or words, or writing of these people is considered to be of the highest value. Note the traditional definition of enlightenment is the absence of Rajas and Tamas in the mind; and that the person has made an effort through penance, austerities, meditation, etc. to achieve knowledge. This knowledge is defined as "continuous or uninterrupted". This means that the Rishi is abiding in a permanent state of knowledge; it is not a transient state of ordinary knowledge that leaves us when we sleep. The Rishi has uninterrupted knowledge of the three states – past, present and future – because they abide in the fourth state called *Turiya*, or that which is beyond the fourth called *Turiyatita*. So according to Indian tradition this kind of knowledge is:

1) Very rare
2) Can be trusted 100%

Definition of Direct Perception:

"The knowledge which that is instantaneously manifest as a result by the proximity of the Jivatman, sense organs, mind, and objects is known as *Pratyaksha* (direct perception)." CS.SU.11.20.

Direct perception is the next best form of knowledge. Note the wording in the Sutra above that says, "knowledge which that is instantaneously...". This is the key wording to the definition of Direct Perception in the Indian tradition. Any knowledge that comes "instantaneously" is not influenced by the conditioned psychology of the person. Hence, any knowledge or information that comes after thinking or reflection is not direct perception because it has been modified by the psychology. Therefore, the meaning of Direct Perception is that it is knowledge that arrives to a Sattvic mind – in other words only a Rishi can have Direct Perception. This is because the nature of Rajas and Tamas is to change and modify anything they come into contact with.

Definition of Inference:

"Inference is preceded by perception. It is of three types and is related to the present, past, and future. For example, fire is inferred from smoke, sexual intercourse from pregnancy; these two belong to the present and past respectively. One can also infer the future fruit from the seed of a tree; this belongs to the inference of the future." CS.SU.11.21-22

Inference is based on perception of an object. Inference is rooted in time, either the present, past or future. Hence, with this form of knowledge we are under the domination of Rajas and Tamas that control the normal human psychology. *This means that the knowledge gained through Inference is subjective because it is modified by the conditioned mind (Manas) and intellect (Buddhi).* Therefore, this kind of knowledge is good, but is not completely reliable. If the psychology is stable then the inferences will be correct. However, many people have disturbed minds, sometimes temporarily, sometimes permanently; these modify the conclusions of inference. For example, saying that Kapha causes dryness is incorrect. But saying that Vata can cause dryness because it dries out Kapha is correct. In this example we know that the Guna of Vata is dryness. By inference we can then see that dryness in the body – in the past, in the future, and in the present – are caused by Vata. It is wrong inference to give this attribute to Kapha, at any time, because it does not have dryness as one of its Gunas.

Definition of Reasoning:

"The intellect which perceives things as the outcome of multiple causative factors, from either the past, present or future, is known as *Yukti* (reasoning). Reasoning helps in the attainment of the three objectives in human life; Dharma, Artha and Kama."
CS.SU.11.25

Reasoning is based on the correct use of the Buddhi or intellect. The intellect is dominated by Rajas and Tamas which are rooted in time, either the present or past or future. These two Maha Gunas (Rajas and Tamas) influence the perception of the object (i.e., patient) and the intellectual process used to arrive at a conclusion concerning the object. *The intellect and reasoning are valuable tools, but they are completely subjective because they are rooted in time and controlled by Rajas and Tamas.* Hence, Reasoning as a means of knowledge is subject to interpretation and manipulation by the psychology of the practitioner. This is unavoidable. The more stable and adaptable the psychology is the better the conclusion will be from the reasoning process. Reasoning is based on the law of cause and effect.

"If seeds are planted at the right time with the right earth and enough water I will have a crop."

This is a logical reasoning process given in the Caraka to show what reasoning is (CS.SU.11.23). Reasoning will give good results if there is a good understanding of the subject. For example, if nothing is known about growing crops then there may not be a successful reasoning outcome to the use of the seeds. *The same is true in Ayurveda; if the practitioner has not memorized anatomy and physiology it will inevitably lead to wrong logic and reasoning.*

Conclusions About Caraka and Gathering Knowledge

The classical method of teaching Ayurveda relies on the Sutras of both Caraka and Susruta as the ultimate authority. This is followed by the teacher who is enlightened. This is followed by the teacher who has lived with an enlightened Rishi or has committed to memory the Caraka and Susruta Samhitas. This is followed by the teacher that has learned from inference and experience. This is followed by the teacher who has learned from reasoning and experience. The last teacher is the least reliable.

Hence, there is a clear hierarchy of ways to acquire knowledge. When applied to Prakriti diagnosis it means the following:
1) We must memorize the attributes and functions of the dosha
2) We should learn to observe the patient with a neutral mind – a mind which is not disturbed by Rajas and Tamas
3) We should practice correct Inference by the study of the Samhitas and by study with a qualified teacher.
4) We should practice correct Reasoning by the study of the Samhitas and by study with a qualified teacher.

All forms of diagnosis are facilitated by a stable mind (psychology). The next lesson expands the subject of Ayurvedic psychology as per Prakriti. Any Prakriti type is capable of obtaining a reasonable diagnosis. Any method that helps attain a clear, stable mental functioning is extremely important. In classical India these methods are Pranayama (observation of breath) and Mantra (repetition of sounds). The regular use these kind of methods improve all metal capacities in all areas of life. When the mind is stable the diagnosis will be more accurate. If the mind of the practitioner is unstable then the diagnosis can be questionable or inaccurate.

In closing the analytical scientific person of today is also prone to the same problems of subjective analysis of data. Any data that is perceived by the five senses and absorbed into the mind will be interpreted subjectively according to the knowledge bias of the scientist. This is a common problem today – when the same data is given to different kinds of scientists they each interpret the data according to their discipline. Hence, the outline that Caraka has given on the collection of data and its interpretation is as valid for Ayurveda as any other science, modern or traditional.

The Nature of the Three Dosha

Observation through the five senses is the most important aspect of diagnosis, as it is more reliable than the patient's own testimony. Caraka gives us a clue as to how to go about observation by reminding us that we have five tools of perception: our five senses.

He writes: "Gather knowledge using the sense organs:
Listen for: gurgling sounds of the intestines, cracking sounds in joints, characters of voice and other body sounds.

Look for: color, shape, size, luster, normal and abnormal characters of the body, etc., and other visual indications.

Taste: should be inferred in this way; inquire about the taste in the patient's mouth by questioning him.

Smell: normal or abnormal smells, in the patient's body.

Touch: normal or abnormal feelings on the hand, or when pressing on the body. CS.VIM.4.7

In Ayurveda the dosha always express their Gunas or attributes. If there is an expression of a Guna then the dosha that is related to that Guna will be there. This true in all levels and applications. For example, Vata will express the same attributes for Prakriti, Vikriti, and in all forms of disease pathology. The dosha do not change their basic attributes or Gunas. Therefore, we use the attributes or Gunas of the dosha to determine which one or which two are dominating the physiology and metabolism; thus indicating Prakriti.

Caraka gives us an idea of how to do this in the following tables (CS.VIM.8.96-99):

Due to this Attribute	Vata Prakriti have these attributes
Dryness	Rough, undeveloped and short body. Long drawn, dry, low, broken, obstructed and hoarse voice, difficulty sleeping
Lightness	Light and unsteady movements (gait), activities, diet and speech
Mobility	Unstable joints, eye brows, jaw, lips, tongue, head, shoulder, hands and feet/legs
Abundance	Talkativeness and abundance of tendons and venous network
Swiftness	Hasty initiation of activities, quick to irritate and quick onset of disorders. Quick in feeling fear, attachment and disenchantment. Quick to learn but quick to forget
Coldness	Intolerance to cold, continuous infliction with cold, shivering and stiffness
Coarseness	Coarse hairs, beard-mustaches, small hairs, nails, teeth, face, hands and feet
Non-sliminess	Cracked body parts, constant sound in joints during movement
	Because of the presence of these qualities, these people have: a lesser degree of strength, life-span, progeny, means and wealth. This whole chart - CS.VIM.8.98

Due to this Attribute	Pitta Prakriti have these attributes
Hotness	Intolerant to heat, having hot face, delicate and fair organs, plenty of moles, freckles, black moles and pimples excessive hunger and thirst, early appearance of wrinkles, graying and falling of hairs, mostly soft, sparse, and brown beard-mustaches
Sharpness	Sharp prowess, intense fire, taking plenty of food and drink, lack of endurance, frequently eating
Liquidity	Lax and soft joints and muscles; secretion of sweat, urine and feces in large quantities
Fleshy smell	Excessive fetid smell, mouth, head and body
Pungency and sourness	Insufficiency of semen, sexual desire and therefore lower progeny
	Because of the presence of all of these qualities, Pitta person having predominance in Pitta are: moderate in strength, life-span, knowledge, understanding, wealth, means. This whole chart - CS.VIM.8.97

Due to this Attribute	Kapha Prakriti have these attributes
Unctuousness	Unctuous organs
Smoothness	Smooth organs
Softness	Pleasing appearance, tenderness and clarity of complexion
Sweetness	Abundant semen, desire and progeny
Firmness	Firmness, compactness and stable of body
Solidity	Plumpness and roundness or all organs
Slowness	Slow in activities, eating, speech, etc.
Rigidity	Resistance in initiating actions
Heaviness	Stable movement with the entire foot pressing against the earth
Coldness	little hunger, thirst, pyrexia (getting hot) and perspiration
Sliminess	Firmness and compactness in the joints / well-united and strong joint ligaments
Clarity	Happiness in the look and face; clear eyes and face with clear and unctuous complexion and affectionate voice.
	Because of the presence of all of these qualities, k persons are: strong, wealthy, learned, brave, calm and long-lived.

These charts are from - CS.VIM.8.96

Basic Protocol to Use to Determine Prakriti

Prakriti is often masked or covered up by imbalanced doshas or Vikriti. This is why the most reliable indicator of Prakriti is the structure and form of the body. Some things like weight, hair color, nails and even skin are modified so much these days that they are not reliable for Prakriti analysis. Depending on the individual these less-reliable characteristics may or may not indicate Prakriti, since Vikriti does not necessarily follow the Prakriti. For example, if there are sufficient Kapha aggravating factors present in our life, we will create a Kapha Vikriti – even if our Prakriti is Vata or Pitta.

All knowledge about Prakriti must represent a life-long pattern of health in order to qualify for Prakriti pariksha. Making observations about structure and form of the body structure, skeleton and tongue are therefore the most reliable indications of Prakriti. Digestion and disease tendency can be used as secondary indications.

Suggested Protocol to Determining Prakriti

Step 1: Physical observations:
1. Face, head & neck (structure and form)
2. Tongue (structure and form)
3. Hands, wrists & arms (structure and form)

Step 2: Questions about metabolism (life-long tendency):
1. Appetite (pattern of hunger)
2. Digestion (nature and imbalance tendency)
3. Elimination (stool, urine and sweat)
4. Circulation (cold hands and feet)
5. Menstruation (for women only)

Step 3: Questions about behavioral and mental traits (life-long tendency):
1. Understanding the motivation behind actions
2. Identifying general behavioral and mental traits

Step 4: Synthesis of parts 1-3.
1. Combine the results from steps 1-3
2. Investigate additional points if required through questioning
3. Make a provisional conclusion of Prakriti

Step 1 - Physical observations (structure and form)

The general rules for interpreting structure and form are as follows:

- **Vata Dosha produces**: long and narrow features, thinness, and irregularity (asymmetric or disproportional features).
- **Pitta Dosha produces**: medium proportions with angular or sharp features, generally quite symmetrical.
- **Kapha Dosha produces**: round, compact, thick, square features, highly symmetrical.

These rules can be applied to observations about the shape (proportions) within the face, the tongue and hands and wrists.

Face diagnosis

Using these rules, we can begin to evaluate the dominant dosha in a person's face:

- Vata shows up as length, thinness, with irregularities and elongated features
- Pitta shows up as medium, well-proportioned, with angular and sharp features
- Kapha shows up as round, square, wide, blunt, thick features

This chart can give some ideas about face shape for different types.

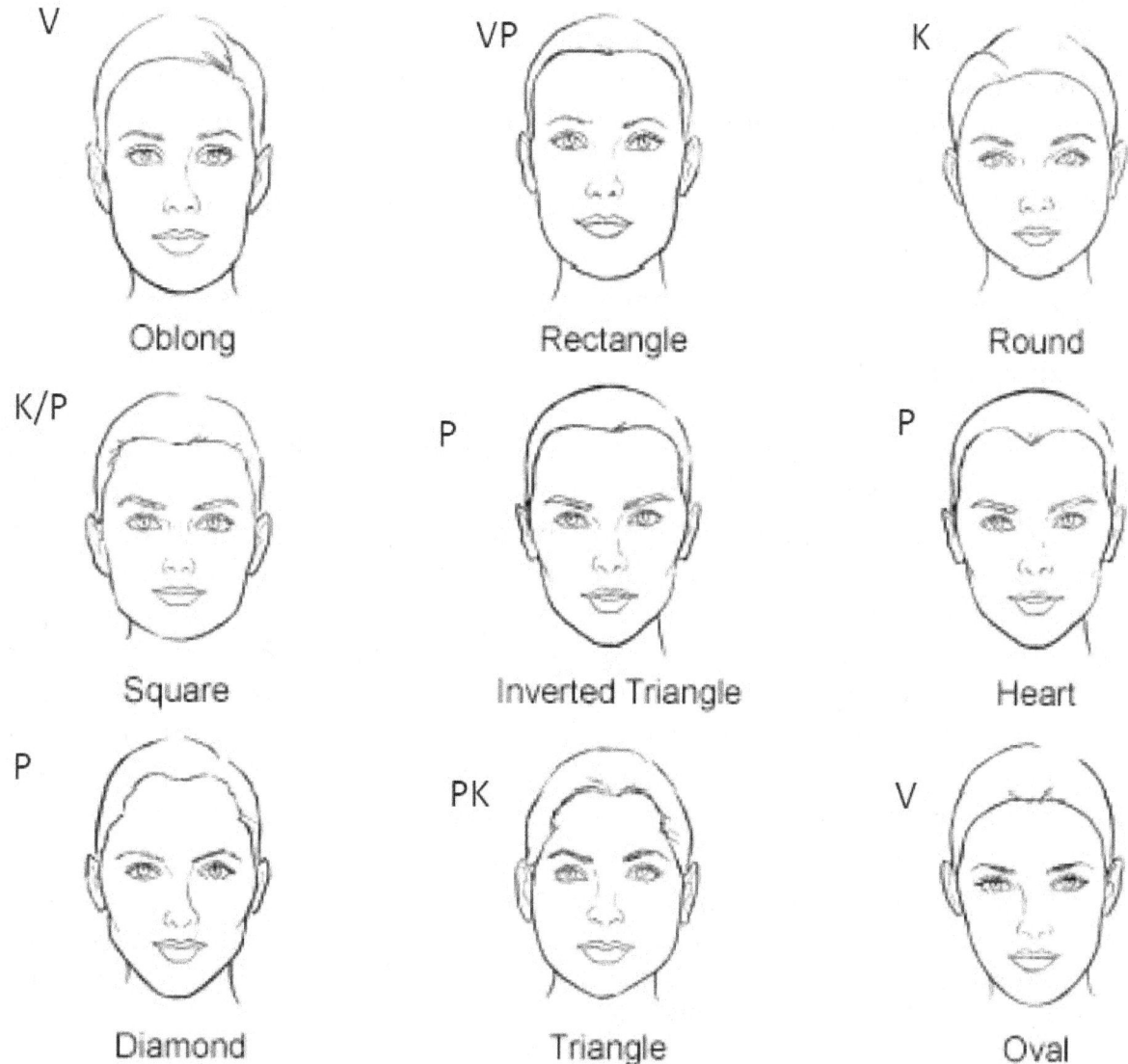

So the overall shape of a Vata face is long and thin. Vata eyes will be relatively small, thin. Vata lips will be thin. Vata ears may stick out, or be hung at slightly different positions. Vata noses are thin, pointed, and perhaps crooked. Vata also causes over-bite and under-bite, as well as crooked, irregular teeth. Vata tends to produce dry, scanty head hair and facial hair.

Pitta produces a medium sized face with slightly angular or sharp features. For example, the eyebrows may be angular, or the chin, or the nose. Pitta lips will be medium sized and well colored. A Pitta nose is medium sized. Pitta often produces less facial hair of a finer nature.

Kapha makes round, wide faces. All the features are rounder, softer, and plumper. Kapha tends to produce thick, voluminous head hair and abundant facial hair (such as eyebrows).

As with all observations, we must be prepared for the dual type Prakriti. By mixing the characteristics of the two doshas, we can arrive at some useful generalizations for the face:

- Vata-Pitta types have a long-to-medium face with some irregularities and some angular features.

- Vata-Kapha types often have a medium sized face with an *absence of angular or sharp features* (that would otherwise tell signs of a Pitta face). Features within the face can either be medium, or long/thin or short/wide/round. Irregularities can be present as well as plump, round features.
- Pitta-Kapha faces are medium-to-wide, solid, with slightly angular and slightly rounded features.

Tongue diagnosis in Prakriti

One of the most reliable diagnosis of Prakriti is to consider the structure and form of the tongue. Even in pathologies, the tongue's shape and form does not change much.

Evaluate the width, length and shape of the tongue. The mouth should be opened as wide as possible without straining, and then the tongue should be slowly extended outwards. It should be extended as far as possible, then retracted until reaching a comfortable position, say about two-thirds extension. Notice how the shape changes as this happens? No matter what the Prakriti, the tongue will become narrower and thicker the more it is extended. So it is important to see the tongue extended and retracted to assess its true shape. The best position general is about two-thirds extended.

When considering the width of the tongue, we must use the lower teeth as a reference point. With the tongue at the two-thirds extended position, compare its width to the mid-line of the teeth. If the tongue appears to be narrower than the teeth, we say it is a *narrow tongue*. If it appears about the same as the teeth (and no more) we say it is a *medium tongue*. If it appears wider than the teeth (especially towards the mid-to-tip end of the tongue) we say it is a *wide tongue*.

The width and shape of the tongue:

- A thin, narrow, pointed tongue indicates Vata Prakriti
- A medium thickness and width tongue indicates Pitta Prakriti
- A thick, wide, round tongue indicates Kapha Prakriti

Remember however that a fully extended tongue will always become narrower and more pointed.

When people have dual type Prakriti the basic rule is to combine the characteristics of the two doshas. Consider the following:

- Vata-Pitta Prakriti, where Vata dominates slightly over Pitta. This can produce a tongue that is narrow-to-medium width, with a steady taper towards a point.
- Pitta-Vata Prakriti, where Pitta dominates slightly over Vata. This can produce a tongue that is medium (like Pitta) but with a pointed tip (from Vata).
- Vata-Kapha Prakriti, this can produce a tongue that is wide (from Kapha) but with a pointed tip (from Vata) and not that thick.

- Pitta-Kapha Prakriti, this can give a normal width, or a wide tongue that is medium thickness.

These are just some ways in which the dual type Prakriti can create a mixed characteristics, in this case the tongue width and shape.

Tongue diagnosis guide (Prakriti)

VATA (narrower than teeth)
Thin, sometimes non-symmetrical, sometimes pointed at the tip, often a matt pinkish color

PITTA (same as teeth)
Medium thickness, sometimes sharp at the tip, often slightly redder than average color

KAPHA (wider than teeth)
Thick, round, usually somewhat blunt, often slightly pale-pink in color

---

Some people say that because Pitta is tikshna (sharp), it can also produce a pointed-tipped tongue. The bottom line in all observational interpretations is that if the observation corresponds to two or more of a dosha's Gunas then is most likely due to that dosha. It is only through the observation of compound attributes that we can become sure of our diagnosis. This is why we must consider several Gunas or characteristics rather than only one in isolation.

Tongue thickness:

- Vata, due to sukshma Guna (subtle/small quality) and laghu Guna (light quality) tends to result in thinness, narrowness, lightness and fineness in all structural situations. Hence Vata Prakriti produces a thin tongue.
- Kapha, due to sthula Guna (gross/big quality) and guru Guna (heavy quality), tends to produce width, thickness, heaviness, roundedness, and bluntness. Hence a Kapha tongue will be the thickest.
- Pitta tongues tend to be in-between Vata and Kapha.

Tongue and general mobility:

- Due to sthira Guna (static quality), Kapha types tend to have quite a solid, immobile tongue. They often have difficulty extending their tongue out of their mouth.
- Vata types tend to have very malleable tongues which come a long way out of the mouth.
- Pitta falls in-between Vata and Kapha.

Tongue color:

All tongues are normally more or less pink. However, depending upon the Prakriti, the tongue color may vary slightly.

- A pinkish-grey or matt tongue indicates Vata Prakriti
- A pinkish-red or dark red tongue Pitta Prakriti
- A pinkish-pale tongue indicates Kapha Prakriti

Tongue color can change in pathologies, but less quickly than other observations.

Hands & Wrists diagnosis in Prakriti

When examining the hands, take note of the overall development of the hand (light, medium, well-built), the overall proportions of the hand (long, medium, square/round), the proportions of the palm (long, medium, square), the proportion of the finger relative to the palm (long, medium or short fingers), the shape of the nails (long, medium or short); in each case, the dosha correspondence is Vata, Pitta, Kapha.

Mixed types show mixed features. Vata-Pitta will show long-medium hands. Pitta-Kapha will show medium to square hands. Vata-Kapha will show medium hands. Be careful with medium hands: they can indicate Pitta or Vata-Kapha Prakriti . If the hands are warm, with a freckly, slightly oily, reddish-ruddy color, they are probably Pitta hands. If they are cold or cool, slightly moist, pale or sallow, then it is probably a Vata-Kapha hand. Vata-Kapha hands can also manifest long palms and fingers that are quite chubby and soft. The most important point is that most of these rules can be broken and that we have to be careful with our interpretation – never losing sight of the intrinsic attributes of the doshas.

As with all observations in Prakriti diagnosis any irregularity or deformity show a dominance of Vata dosha. So hands, which despite their other characteristics, that show up some blatant irregularities must be considered as belonging to a pure or mixed Vata Prakriti. Even when the hands seem unusually small or large in proportion to the rest of the body.

Hands diagnosis guide (Prakriti)

VATA (long)	**PITTA (medium)**	**KAPHA (compact)**
Long and thin, disproportional (fingers relative to palms), long palms, brittle nails	Medium build, well proportioned, medium-rectangular palms, soft nails	Compact-thick build, symmetrical (fingers and palms similar length), hardy nails

---

In addition to the face, tongue and hands, there are other considerations of physical observations; such as the overall skeletal structure. A thin frame with long limbs indicates Vata. A medium frame indicates Pitta, and a more compact, well-build frame with shorter limbs indicates Kapha. No matter where the dosha are they always will manifest or express their attributes. Thus, the structure – no matter where it is in the body – will show the dominate dosha's attributes. To understand the body structure as a whole it can be easier to use the questionnaire that is found at the end of this lesson.

Step 2 – Metabolic Diagnosis in Prakriti

The most *reliable* indications of Prakriti are found in the structure and form of the body. These things do not vary too much with age or illnesses. All other metabolic indicators (such as appetite or menstruation) are subject to change and so require a more cautious approach when used for Prakriti pariksha. The overall metabolic nature of a person is a direct reflection of the function of Jathar Agni which is regulated by the three dosha. When we begin to examine the various metabolic indicators, we must always validate our findings by asking if they represent the *lifelong pattern of the patient*. If there is doubt then less emphasis should be placed on the findings. For example, someone might have had irregular hunger patterns, digestion and elimination since the age of 25 when they had a car accident, but these qualities could easily have been caused by the trauma which put Vata dosha into a perpetual state of aggravation. Prior to this time, the appetite and digestion might have been regular. Failure to check the temporal nature of the metabolic observations leads to mistakes in the diagnosis of Prakriti . The following are some of the most important indicators of the metabolic nature: appetite, elimination, circulation and menstruation for women.

Tendencies of Digestive Problems and Metabolic Malfunctions

These are some of the most common signs that each constitution is out of equilibrium. This indicates that the metabolism is not functioning correctly. A patient does not have to experience all of these symptoms at once. Any symptom, if consistent, will indicate some degree of metabolic disturbance. The following indications are not health, but they do indicate the Prakriti by the disease tendency.

Vata Type Malfunctions Common to Vata Prakriti people :

Gas, constipation, colic pain, gripping, dry stools, bloating abdomen, PMS, dry skin or hair, nervousness, anxiety, insomnia, aversion to cold weather and wind, food allergies, and irregularity in occurrence of any of these symptoms.

Pitta Type Malfunctions Common to Pitta Prakriti people :

Burning in the stomach or abdomen, loose stools, ulcers, inflamed intestines, hemorrhoids, skin inflammation, burning eyes, headaches that are light sensitive, aversion to heat, irritation or frustration.

Kapha Type Malfunctions Common to Kapha Prakriti people :

Nausea, bloating in the stomach, congestion in the lungs or stomach, feeling of heaviness, difficulty to get motivated, desire to eat frequently, aversion to damp and cold, depression, craving for sweets and food allergies.

The Ayurvedic view of the metabolism is that it strives for equilibrium naturally. The metabolism achieves equilibrium through the three dosha. **Imbalance of Dosha tends to follow the constitution, which is a reflection of the dominate Dosha.** Therefore, the Vata type will tend to show the signs of Vata attributes in a state of metabolic disturbance. The Pitta type will tend to show signs of Pitta attributes in a state of disturbance, and the Kapha type will tend to show signs of Kapha attributes in a state of disturbance.

Appetite Evaluation

Each Prakriti type controls Agni in a different manner. The appetite is a direct reflection of the function or state of Agni and Agni is a result of dosha dominance. The following table illustrates this:

One way to judge the appetite of the patient is to ask at what time hungry starts in the morning. Pitta dosha governs Agni in general through the function of Pachaka Pitta. The Doshas are modified by the movement of time – this concept is explained in the section on

Appetite evaluation in Prakriti Pariksha		
Prakriti	Agni tendency	Appetite tendency
Vata	Variable High or Low	Erratic appetite, quick to become hungry, quick to satisfy, small capacity, variable hungry, can miss meals, can forget to eat.
Pitta	High Excessive, Regular	Strong, sometimes excessive appetite, needs large meals, large capacity, needs three meals per day, does not miss meals.
Kapha	Low Insufficient, Regular	Low appetite, often eats due to habit, appetite less in the morning, eats emotionally, can skip a meal.
Vata-Pitta	Variable to High Sometimes variable Sometimes excessive	Erratic appetite depending on which dosha is the strongest, moderate capacity though can vary, needs to eat often, can feel weak or irritated if meals are late or missed
Vata-Kapha	Variable to Low, Sometimes variable Sometimes low	Erratic appetite, depending on which dosha is the strongest, low capacity, quick to satisfy, sometimes needs to eat, eats emotionally
Pitta-Kapha	High to Low Regular Sometimes high Sometimes low	Strong, consistent appetite, though usually appetite is moderate and regular, capacity is large, can eat emotionally, skipping a meal may be possible, less hungry in the morning

pathology. This vision states that each Dosha goes through a natural cycle of increasing, becoming aggravated and decreasing. This cycle is reflected in the movement of time; time of day and season the year. According to this thought the morning is Kapha time of the day. This means that the attributes of Kapha manifest strongly at this time. Hence, Kapha Prakriti types will have a delayed onset of hunger since the qualities of Kapha are dominate at that time of day. The opposite will apply to Pitta Prakriti types as they do not have Kapha attributes in their body to the same extent. The following chart illustrates how each Prakriti typology will tend to become hungry in the morning.

Assuming that the subject wakes up between 6am and 10am (6h to 10h):

Appearance of hunger for Prakriti pariksha	
Prakriti	Onset of hunger
Vata	1 to 2 hours after waking
Pitta	30 minutes to 1 hour after waking
Kapha	3 to 4 hours after waking
Vata-Pitta	1 to 1.5 hours after waking
Vata-Kapha	1.5 to 2.5 hours after waking
Pitta-Kapha	2 to 3 hours after waking

Using these two guides, it is possible to assess the life-long hunger pattern. Note that besides *dosha vriddhi* (excess dosha), there are a few things that can distort the above table:

- **Ama** – If toxins are present in the intestines, they will soon cause reduced appetite for all types. It can be Ama that causes a chronic lack of appetite in the mornings – this will be covered under the section on pathology.

- **Age** – Children and teenagers have a relatively strong appetite. The opposite happens in old age as Vata dosha increases, the appetite tends to diminish gradually.

- **Gender** – Men tend to have bigger appetites than women.

- **Body size** – A general rule is that the bigger the person, the bigger their stomach. Usually the stomach size is related to appetite.

- **Occupation & general level of activity** – Appetite normally depends on the level of activity. The more physical exercise there is the more an appetite will develop. The inverse is also true. This means that if a young, pure Kapha type is working at a very physical job, they may well develop an appetite that is strong in the early morning.

- **Cultural differences** – Some countries have a tradition of eating a big breakfast, like in the USA, for example. The French on the other hand enjoy a much lighter continental breakfast. Thus, cultural conditioning can modify the eating habits of the individual. A French Pitta type may be less likely to be hungry at breakfast than an American one, whereas an American Kapha might be less likely to accept not eating breakfast than a French one.

Elimination Evaluation

After judging the appetite, the elimination is the next most important indicator of Agni function.

Mixed types show mixed signs, depending on which dosha is dominant, or simply by mixing the indications together. Like hunger, elimination can be adversely affected by certain factors other than basic dosha aggravation. Some of these are:

- A diet high in refined foods and animal protein is heavy to digest which creates a sluggish elimination. This is most true for Vata and Kapha types, and less true for Pitta types.
- A course of antibiotics can disturb the balance of positive bacteria in the colon, resulting in bloating, gas, constipation or other disturbances.
- Certain medications provoke constipation and even food supplements such as iron.

Here are the general patterns for Prakriti types.

Elimination tendency for Prakriti	
Prakriti	**Elimination tendency**
Vata	Vata types tend to have variable elimination. When healthy, they will eliminate 1-2 times a day and the stool will be well formed. There is a tendency towards having dry, hard, medium colored, irregular and scanty stools. The stool can be in several pieces. Vata types have the least smelly stool. If the stool is hard there can be cramping pain in the lower left abdomen prior to elimination and evacuation can be uncomfortable.
Pitta	Pitta types tend to have frequent elimination. When healthy, they will eliminate between 1-2 times a day in large amounts and the stool will be well formed. There is a tendency towards loose stools, or the stool breaking into 2-3 parts. Pitta types have stronger smelling stool due to their fiery nature and control of bile, and their stool tends to be darker than the other types. A pure Pitta type will never be constipated.
Kapha	Kapha types tend to have sluggish elimination. When healthy, they will eliminate once a day and the stool will be well formed. There is a tendency towards congestion or constipation. The stool tends towards being sticky, light colored and moderate in quantity. Kapha types have the slowest digestion and elimination, but remain regular. They may need time in the morning to eliminate the stool.

It is important to look for lifelong tendencies of digestion and elimination. The tendency of imbalance is usually a good indicator of Prakriti.

Circulation Evaluation

Another metabolic tool for determining Prakriti is blood circulation.

Blood Circulation for Prakriti	
Prakriti	**Blood Circulation tendency**
Vata	Vata types tend to have poor, variable circulation. They have the least resistance to the climate changes and are effected by cold more than any type. They often suffer from cold hands and feet.
Pitta	Pitta types have good circulation. They may need to have their feet hanging out of bed at night. They often have sweating hands and feet. They resist cold well, but often cannot function well in hot climates.
Kapha	Kapha types have a slow circulation. They often have cool hands and feet, though a good resistance to climate changes in general. They are prone to congestive problems in circulation.

Menstruation Evaluation

For women the menstrual cycle is a valuable tool for Prakriti evaluation. It is, perhaps, the single most important indicator of Prakriti because it is a direct reflection of metabolic processes and a woman's health in general.

Several factors should be considered in the menstrual cycle. The *timing* of the menstrual cycle and the *quality* and *quantity* of the menstrual blood itself. Timing of all bodily processes is governed by Vata Dosha. Vata tends to function quickly, Pitta is average, and Kapha is slow in function. Therefore, Vata types tend to have the shortest menstrual bleeding of 2 – 3 days, Pitta types average with 3 – 5 days, and Kapha types the longest with 4 – 7 day cycles. However, when the menstruation lasts more than 7 days, it is a sign that the metabolism is disturbed. In terms of the menstrual blood itself, this is considered to be under the domain of Kapha and Pitta doshas. Kapha because menstrual fluid is the upadhatu of Rasa Dhatu. Pitta because it controls the uterus and vagina which are part of Rakta Dhatu.

Dual constitutions will have mixed indications before and during menstruation. More precise detail on the nature of menstruation can be found in my book on women's health *"Ayurvedic Healing for Women"*. In this book there are detailed descriptions of different Prakriti combinations and tendencies.

Menstrual tendency for Prakriti	
Prakriti & Cycle	**Menstrual tendency**
Vata 26-28 day cycle	Short menstruation is normal (2–3 days). Vata types have the lightest menstruation, but are the most prone to Premenstrual Syndrome difficulties. Before and during the first day of bleeding they can have fatigue, cramping or throbbing headaches. Blood may be dark with a small quantity of fluid due the dryness of Vata. Irregular cycles, delayed menstruation and strong PMS can all indicate Vata aggravation.
Pitta 28 day cycle	Medium duration is normal (3–5 days). Pitta types have the heaviest blood loss during menstruation. They are the most prone very heavy bleeding with heavy blood loss leading to anemia, fatigue and low energy. Blood may be bright red with clots. Loose stools, irritability and burning headaches can all indicate Pitta aggravation.
Kapha 28-30 day cycle	Longer duration is normal (4–7 days). Kapha types have a medium flow. They are the least prone to PMS symptoms although they can become the most emotional before and during menstruation. The fluid is lighter in color and has a thicker consistency than other types. There can be clots in the fluid. Dull aching pain, dull headaches and the feeling to cry can all indicate Kapha aggravation.

Conclusions on Body Constitution or Prakriti

The physical and metabolic analysis should reflect the body's Prakriti. The classic teaching is that the body and mind will have the same Prakriti. The next lessons address the mental or psychological aspect of Prakriti.

Different doctors have different methods of codifying their findings during and after diagnosis. There is no standard way to do this in Ayurveda. Some practitioners use charts, numbers or graphs. I personally prefer a graph without a numerical value because I am sensitive to numerical classifications of unique human beings. This approach is presented later in disease diagnosis. Any method that works for the practitioner is acceptable. Patients often want "to know what their Prakriti is" so expect some kind of numeric, or other evaluation. In this case a simple chart like the one below can be used. Here is a hypothetical evaluation:

	Vata	Pitta	Kapha
Tongue	1	1	
Faces	1		
Hands		1	
Skeleton	1		
Appetite	1	1	
Digestion			1
Elimination	1		
Circulation		1	
Menstruation	1		1
Totals	**6**	**4**	**2**

For example, the tongue may have a Vata – Pitta form. With two scores at Vata = 6 and Pitta = 4, this person would be classified as a Vata-Pitta Prakriti awaiting verification through treatments. If the score was Vata = 7, Pitta = 3, Kapha = 1, then it would indicate a pure Vata Prakriti .

Many practitioners prefer to use a constitutional analysis test or questionnaire. I have made a questionnaire that I feel is far superior to other similar exams for one basic reason: Prakriti and Vikriti are clearly separated for the patient. This avoids the major pitfall of constitutional analysis hat confuses lifetime (Prakriti) tendencies with temporary or disease (Vikriti) tendencies. The advantage of this kind of questionnaire is that it is detailed and gives an insight into the many indications of Prakriti. The disadvantage is that it takes time to fill out correctly.

Look over the questionnaire below and choose either Vata - 'V', Pitta - 'P', or Kapha - 'K' for each category. Choose one answer per category, do not choose two answers. For each answer there are two answer columns – the lifetime tendencies (Prakriti) and the present tendencies (Vikriti). This means for each category there will be one response for 'lifetime' and one response for 'present'. An example of this could be for the category of 'Body

Weight' I might put 'P' as the answer for the 'lifetime' column and 'K' as the answer for the 'present' column if I had suddenly begun to gain weight in the last 2 or 3 years.

Once the questionnaire is finished total up the numbers of V's, P's and K's. Whatever Dosha has the highest score will indicate the constitution and the imbalance. If two types are very close to being the same amount consider the person to be a mixed or dual type. An example of this could be a score of 14 – V, 12 – P, and 5 – K. This would show a dual or mixed type of Vata-Pitta. Generally a range of plus or minus 4 points indicates a dual type of person.

CATEGORY	LIFETIME	PRESENT
Body Frame		
V-tall or short, thin, poorly developed physique P-medium height, moderately developed physique K-stout, stocky, big, well developed physique		
Body Weight		
V-light, hard to hold weight P-moderate weight K-heavy, gains weight easily		
Skin Texture		
V-dry, rough or cracked, prominent veins P-moist, pink, freckles K-white, moist, soft		
Skin Temperature		
V-cold P-warm K-cool		
Hair Quality		
V-coarse, dry, split ends P-fine, soft, can grey or bald early K-abundant, oily, thick, lustrous		
Face Shape		
V- small, thin, long P-medium sized, oval K-large, round, fat		
Teeth		
V- often crooked P- medium sized K- large, even		
Gums		
V- dark, receding gums P- red, gums bleed easily K- soft, pink		
Tongue Width		
V-narrower than teeth, long and thin P-same width as teeth, oval shaped front K-wider than teeth, thick, round front		
Quality of Hands		
V-fine, dry, cold, long fingers P-symmetrical, pink, warm K-large, thick and short fingers		

Finger Nails		
V-thin, rough, fissured, cracked, darkish P-strong, pinkish K-thick, smooth, white		
Digestive Strength		
V-variable or weak, often has allergies P-strong, able to digest most anything K-medium or slow but steady		
Digestive Disturbances		
V-intestinal gas P-acidity or burning K-bloated feeling or heaviness, nausea		
Food Attractions		
V-dry, sweet or salty, crispy snack foods P-spicy, salty, hot K-sweet, creamy, cold		
Food Habits		
V-binges, snacks, forgets to eat P-likes regular, plentiful meals K-eats constantly, overeats regularly		
Food Sensitivities		
V-beans, cabbage family P-onions, tomatoes, fried foods K-dairy, salt		
Urination		
V-two to four times per day P-four to six times per day K-three to five times per day		
Feces		
V-dry, hard, difficult or painful, gas, tends towards constipation P-abundant, loose, sometimes yellowish, tends towards diarrhea K-moderate, solid, sometimes pale in color or can have mucus in stool		
Sweat and Body Odor		
V-little with no smell P-profuse, hot, strong smell K-moderate, neutral smell		
Blood Circulation		
V-poor, variable, cold hands & feet P-good, warm hands & feet K-slow but steady, cool hands & feet		

Appetite		
V-variable, erratic P-strong K-constant		
Activities		
V-quick, fast, erratic, hyperactive P-motivated, purposeful, goal seeking K-slow, steady, methodical		
Strength and Endurance		
V- poor endurance, starts & stops P- moderate level of endurance K-strong, good endurance, slow in starting		
Sensitivity to Environment		
V-dislike of cold, wind, sensitive to dryness, likes warmth P-dislike of heat or direct sun, likes coolness K-dislike of cold, damp, likes wind and sun		
Resistance to Disease		
V-poor, variable, weak immune system P-medium, prone to infections K-good, consistent, strong immune system		
Disease Tendency		
V-nervous system diseases, pain, mental disorders, insomnia, eating disorders, arthritis P-febrile diseases, ulcers, infections, inflammatory diseases, heart attacks K-respiratory system diseases, mucus, edema, obesity, benign tumors		
Speech Habits		
V-quick, talkative, inconsistent, erratic P-moderate, argumentative, convincing K-slow, concise, not talkative		
Mental Nature		
V-quick, adaptable, indecisive, impulsive P-factual, penetrating, critical K-slow, steady		
Emotional Response		
V-quick, but soon over P-hot, irritated or defensive, grudge K-slow, but bothers for a long time		
Emotional Tendencies		
V-anxious, fearful, nervous, worries P-frustrated, irritable, angry, dominating K-calm, attached, greedy, sentimental		

Social Relations		
V-relates easy, can be superficial P-relates well, can be dominating K-relates with difficulty		
Mental Relations to Objects		
V-not very important, erratic P-important to know about, purposeful K-important to have or own, practical		
Relationship to Money		
V-not very important P-useful to gain control or respect K-very important		
Relationship to Spending Money		
V-spends easily P-spends for a purpose K-spends with difficulty		
Friends		
V-has many, but not deep P-has close relationships K-has few, but very deep		
Love Relationships		
V-tends to have many, erratic P-tends to marry for position or looks K-single partner, very faithful		
Neurotic Tendencies		
V-hysteria, anxiety attacks, depression P-extreme temper, rage, tantrums K-sorrow, unresponsiveness, depressive, grief		
Life Goals		
V-changing frequently, not so important P-determined, very important K-fixed for life early		
Sleep		
V-light, tends towards insomnia, restless P-moderate, may wake up but will fall asleep again K-heavy, difficulty in waking up in the morning		
TOTALS	V P K	V P K
Lifetime Constitution - Prakriti		
Present Constitution - Vikriti		

Study Questions for Chapter Eleven

1. What are the four sources of knowledge According to Caraka?

2. What are the reliable signs of Prakriti?

3. When can we use metabolic indications as a reliable sign of Prakriti?

4. What are the metabolic indications for people with dual Prakriti?

5. What are the long-term elimination habits for Vata-Pitta Prakriti types?

6. Which type of people are hungry at about 10 am in the morning?

7. Which type of people can gain weight easily?

8. Why is the best indication of Prakriti the structure and form of the body?

9. How far should the tongue be extended to make an accurate observation of Prakriti?

10. Which Prakriti type can be harder to diagnose?

CHAPTER TWELVE
PRAKRITI PARIKSHA - EVALUATION OF MENTAL PRAKRITI

This chapter continues with the next steps in Prakriti Pariksha:

Step 3: Questions about behavioral and mental traits (life-long tendency):

Evaluation of the psychology in Ayurveda rests on the concept that was explained in Chapter Ten; the physical body provides the structure in which the mind functions. See the diagram below that illustrates how the Doshas dominating the body influence the psychology as a whole.

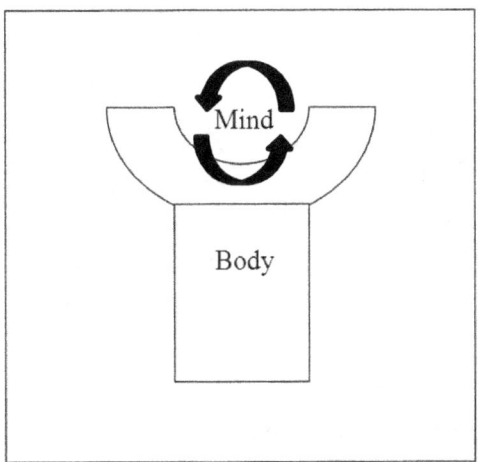

The mental Prakriti is a reflection of the physical Prakriti in terms of the "structure" of the mind. In order to be totally accurate the mind actually manifests first in the Samkhya Darshana and thus establishes an energetic blueprint in the Tanmatra level of creation for the physical body to manifest; this where the three doshas manifest. Hence, if we accept the Vedic vision that pure consciousness becomes progressively encased in matter, then we must also accept that the psychological manifestation is responsible for the manifestation of the physical Prakriti and not the other way around.

Ayurveda is first and foremost a functional vision of medicine. This being the case the functional aspect of the psychology is responsible for the general behavioral and mental traits exhibited by any individual. In Ayurvedic medicine the mind is not the domain of the Doshas – it is the domain of the three Maha Gunas, or Sattva, Rajas and Tamas. This chapter looks in detail at the functional nature of the mind and how it is controlled by the three Gunas. This means that the three Maha Gunas are responsible for the Dosha manifestations and the physical body's manifestation. In the ultimate sense the Maha Gunas determine the Prakriti; physical and mental.

This does not mean that the doshas do not have any effect on the mind and psychology as a whole; they do have an effect. In the diagram above we see the functional mind resting in the structure of the body. This is like putting milk in a copper pot, or milk in an iron pot. The liquid (milk) will take on the characteristics of the vessel holding it. It is not possible to have a mind without a body; the body supports the mind. Thus, when analyzing the Mental Prakriti we should first look at the Dosha dominance in the body. Then we can see the Dosha's twenty Gunas operating in the mind which in turn influences the functional nature of the mind.

This is a more detailed explanation of the mind and psychology generally than is usually given. This explanation is not simplistic and neither is the view expressed by classical texts like the Caraka Samhita. This is explained further in a chapter on clinical psychology presented in Volume Two in this series of textbooks.

There are two important considerations:
1. Understanding the motivation behind actions
2. Identifying general behavioral and mental traits

The motivation of mental actions should evaluated before evaluating the actions themselves. From a functional point of view the "movement" of the mind is more important than the "content" of the mind. Movement we can translate in the psychology as the "intention behind the action". This reveals the dominate Dosha through its Gunas and attributes. The "content" of the mind is more related to conditioning and behavioral traits.

These are fundamental motivating factors for each Dosha:

- Where change and stimulation motivate   – Vata is the reason
- Where achievement or the pursuit of goals motivate – Pitta is the reason.
- Where security, stability or comfort motivate   – Kapha is the reason.

The doshas, through their twenty Gunas, motivate our actions. It is the *intention* behind the action that reveals the true motivating dosha, not the action itself. The following basic drives that arise from each of the doshas:
- Vata is motivated by a desire for change and stimulation. This comes from Vata's light, mobile nature.
- Pitta is motivated by a desire for achievement & recognition. This comes from Pitta's sharp, hot, intense nature.
- Kapha is motivated by a desire for security & stability. This comes from Kapha's slow, heavy, steady nature.

When evaluating the psychology according to Ayurveda the above factors are the most important. They give the indications of which Dosha is dominating because they provide a clue to the real motivations that we have as people. As in the previous lesson we, as practitioners, need to be aware of our own Prakriti bias when evaluating the mind and the motivations behind the psychology as a whole. As with the physical body the mind tends to project itself on to the patient and – without effort – tries to judge the patient's mind with its own mental conditioning. Hence, trying to discover the motivation behind actions is an important way to reduce the Prakriti bias in mental evaluations.

In the introduction of Prakriti in Chapter Ten basic psychological traits have been listed for each of the pure types. This is additional information that shows how the doshas function in the mind:

- Vata dosha is the principle of movement. It is responsible for the movement of thought, and for our basic mental energy. Vata brings things to our attention and governs the mobile, changeable, creative nature of thought and emotions. It allows the five senses to receive information from outside the body and brings it into the conditioned mind (Manas).

- Pitta dosha is the principle of transformation and governs mental digestion. Pitta governs perception, understanding, comprehension and insight. It allows the fire of perception to animate the intellect (Buddhi) and the conditioned mind (Manas).

- Kapha dosha is the principle of cohesion and governs mental stability. It is responsible for our capacity for retention, memory, patience, and perseverance. Kapha allows for a correct mental function because it lubricates and supports the structure that Vata and Pitta are using. In terms of memory it relates to the subconscious mind (Chita).

According to the information above these factors cause the Doshas to function in the following manner:

Vata

An urge to discover new things, explore the unknown and go beyond existing boundaries and the limits of conformity. This pursuit requires Vata to have and use abundant energy. Therefore, anyone who lives for change, stimulation and a love of newness (new things, new ideas, new approaches to life) is probably a Vata type or mixed Vata type Prakriti mentally. The other aspect of Vata is their creative urges. It is difficult for Vata not to create on some level; the expression of newness, the discovery of some new form, shape or color is an important expression of Vata.

Pitta

People who are happiest when working towards clear goals that challenge their expertise and bring the rewards of recognition and a sense of personal achievement are usually Pitta types or a dual Pitta type Mental Prakriti. Their quick, sharp, fiery attributes that come from fire help to perceive and solve problems. Pitta dominant people often find themselves able to achieve and accomplish things that other types are not able to even imagine.

Kapha

People who live for the well-being of others, with strong community and family oriented drives are usually Kapha types or a dual Kapha type Mental Prakriti. They can strive in a steady, methodical way to create more and more security and stability for themselves and their family. This sort of behavior comes from Kapha doshas stability and basic desire for security. People with Kapha dominant Prakriti often feel compelled to keep the status quo which helps them maintain the goal of security.

Mixed or Dual Types

Dual types will show a blend of the pure traits psychologically. There is not fixed rule to understand how the dual types will blend together. Some people will show more of one side and others will show a perfect blending of both Doshas.

Conclusion

The mental Prakriti is influenced by the dominate Dosha that control the form and structure of the body. This influence will cause some basic motivational traits to manifest in the psychology of the patient. Depending on the twenty Guna manifestation of these traits the Dosha will be determined.

Motivational impulses are better guides to Prakriti than actions or psychological conditioning. Therefore, we should try to understand the intentions of people rather than just observing their behavior. Behavior analysis will be covered under the appropriate lesson which goes into the subject of Maha Guna dominance (see the next chapter), or the functional aspect of the psychology. This is less indicative of the Mental Prakriti because it is completely dependent on the nature of the conditioning received during childhood.

Step 4: Synthesis of Physical and Mental Prakriti.

Once the practitioner has made the analysis of the first three steps it is possible to combine these into a working model.

When establishing Prakriti one aspect is not more important than another. First, we should see what is *accurate* – that could the metabolism, it could be the mind, or it could be the form and structure. Each patient will be different and none will have the same accuracy in terms of which will be the most reliable to demonstrate Prakriti.

So rather than always relying on form and structure we *should rely on what is most accurate for that person.* There is no way to avoid subjectivity. Our goal is to reduce the subject factors as much as possible by awareness of the problem. That being said there needs to be a value judgment on what aspect of the person is the most accurate and reliable. Be aware of evaluation bias as discussed in the sections on Prakriti evaluation. Take action to consciously avoid any bias when possible.

If all things seem equally accurate then:

1. Structure and Form
2. Metabolic Functions
3. Mental Motivations

Each can be given one-third importance in establishing the Prakriti of the person.

The best situation for the practitioner is when all three areas of evaluation are equally accurate. This allow us to give one-third importance to each aspect of the Prakriti. This approach gives the most accurate evaluation of the person's Prakriti. If different areas give different Doshas then it will tend to indicate dual or mixed types.

Investigate additional points if required through questioning

If any point is not clear additional questions can be asked at any time by the practitioner. I often go back and ask questions on some point that may have not been clear later on, or even in another appointment.

If a practitioner is insecure it can cause them to be timid to re-question, or clarify points with the patient. On the other hand this same insecurity can manifest as an overly aggressive questioning that intimidates the patient. Clarify any point that is needed concerning the Prakriti Diagnosis, but do so in a respectful manner.

Make a provisional conclusion of Prakriti

To make a conclusion with conflicting data is the most challenging. This gets easier with practice. I often tell my patients that I am not sure of their Prakriti and that I will become clear through observing the response they have with my treatment. Once they understand that the Prakriti is "cover up" by the Vikriti then this explanation is accepted.

Imagine that we have the following results:

Form a Structure:	Pitta – Kapha
Metabolism function:	Pitta – Vata
Mental Evaluation:	Kapha – Vata

This would be about the worst possible result because each Dosha has two indications. In this situation a *qualitative* judgment needs to be made on which evaluation was the most accurate. If this is not possible then tell the patient you will not know until after giving them a treatment and waiting to see which Dosha comes out dominate.

There is nothing wrong with not knowing! There is something wrong with telling people a conclusion that you are not sure about. It is possible to get into real problems by telling a patient they have one type, and then later as the therapies give results, discovering that they are another type. What to do now? Admit a mistake? Try to cover up with fancy Sanskrit terms?

These kinds of problems can be avoided by telling the patients that:
1. Prakriti Analysis is an ongoing observation
2. Treatments are the best confirmation of Prakriti
3. Vikriti is so strong most traces of the Prakriti as not showing
4. And thus, I do not know your Prakriti!

If you think you know the Prakriti, well and good. No problem. Just be aware that is perfectly fine not to know the Prakriti definitively; in fact it is common when the patient is chronically ill.

Study Questions for Chapter Twelve

1. Why is Vata dosha the Dosha that receives outside impressions into the mind?

2. Which of the following reasons motivate Vata types to travel?

3. Which of the following reasons motivate Pitta types to travel?

4. Which of the following reasons motivate Kapha types to travel?

5. What is most likely to cause a Pitta type to become seriously depressed?

6. Why do Vata types tend to forget to eat when they are busy?

7. Why do Pitta types tend to stay focused on their current project?

8. Why do Kapha types tend to be methodical in most activities even if they do not like them?

9. When establishing Prakriti which aspect is the most important?

10. When all Dosha are equal in Prakriti evaluation what will you tell the patient?

CHAPTER THIRTEEN
THE THREE MAHA GUNA & MENTAL PRAKRITI

As we learned in the previous lesson the mental Prakriti is a result of the physical Prakriti because the physical body provides the location for the mind to function. The mental Prakriti has two aspects to it:

1) The relation to the physical Prakriti
2) The functional aspect that works within the body/mind structure

This chapter is concerned with the second aspect, or the functional mind. In many respects this is also the part of our mind that is conditioned by parents, family, education, culture and religion. But it is not limited to this conditional aspect alone. This section explains the relationship between your conditioned mental disposition and your mental Prakriti in terms of the three Gunas / doshas.

Before going into this subject it is important to note two quotes from the Caraka Samhita:

"The Jiva is devoid of all pathology. *He is the cause of consciousness through the mind and senses. He is eternal and the observer of all activities."*
CS.SU.1.56

"Pathogenic factors in the body are vayu, Pitta and Kapha, **while those in the mind are rajas and Tamas."**
CS.SU.1.57

These quotes are from the first chapter of the *Sutrastana* section and establish the foundation of health and disease for Ayurveda as a medical system. The first sutra number fifty-six states that our essence, or Beingness, the Jivatman, is healthy and has no pathology associated with it. The second sutra number fifty-seven states that two of the three Maha Gunas, Rajas and Tamas, cause pathology in the mind.

This means that the functional aspect of the mind or that which functions within the body – our psychology – is NOT the mental Prakriti per se. It is more related to disease factors (Vikriti) than Prakriti. What about the other Guna, Sattva? Why has Caraka not listed

185

Sattva Guna as a disease causing factor? We find the explanation to this question in Sutrastana, Chapter Eight:

"Mind transcends all sense perceptions. It is known as Sattva. ....."
CS.SU.8.4

This sutra is very important because it establishes a definition of the mind. It says that the mind, or human psychology, is prior to any sense perception from the external world and transcends the senses. In other words it exists before the senses and is not the result of sense perception – rather it is the cause of perception. This sutra also establishes the definition of the psychology (Manas) as Sattvic by nature and therefore healthy.

By an analysis of the sutras 1.57 and 8.4 we arrive at two conclusions:
1) Sattva = health
2) The mind = Sattva

Note that in Sanskrit the word "Manas" can mean the mind in general – the psychology – or it can mean one specific part of the mind that is conditioned by its association to the five senses and external world. This means that the mind in general, or the psychology, is healthy and balanced by nature; Sattva. However, it also means that the conditioned part of the mind (Manas), the subconscious mind (Chitta), the intellect (Buddhi) and the sense of "I" or ego (Ahamkara) are prone to disease or mental pathologies due the influence of Rajas and Tamas Gunas.

In simple terms this means that the mind is pure and healthy before the conditioning and interaction with life as a baby, child, adolescence and adult. This is the definition of the mind in Chapter Eight, Sutra Four that says the mind is Sattva. In the other sutra we learn that the other two Maha Gunas Rajas and Tamas cause mental illness or distress, basically from social conditioning.

Hence, the Sattva mind or pure psychology is part of the mental Prakriti. The conditioned mind creates problems because it "covers" this pure (Sattva) mind with action (rajas) and obscurity (Tamas). Thus, the word *Vikriti* literally means *"that which covers Prakriti"*. This is translated as disease, imbalance or pathology as it covers our nature, which according to Ayurveda is health.

Nevertheless, knowing this we cannot ignore the conditioned part of the mind completely when doing the Prakriti mental analysis. We must also judge the levels of the Gunas in the mind and try to understand the basic conditioning of the person in other to judge correctly their overall mental Prakriti. A failure to do this would result in a superficial approach to Ayurveda; or even the vulgarization of Ayurveda. This would reduce it from a global system of medicine, or a body / mind / soul form of medicine, to a mechanical, judgemental system that compartmentalizes people. Therefore, we, as therapists, need to look at the totality of the mind with an objective view to understand how much – to what extent – the pure, Prakriti mind (Sattva) has been covered over by social conditioning. This, of course, is not an easy task.

The first point to make is that 'normal' people (you and I) are all somewhat Rajasic and Tamasic psychologically because our society is basically Rajasic and Tamasic. This is normal that we reflect our society and culture because they are responsible for conditioning our minds as children; and by extension the minds of our parents, grandparents, and so on. In theory, if the culture were Sattvic in nature our minds would remain Sattvic.

Another important point to make before going further in this chapter is the concept of the three Maha Gunas in nature (Samkhya) and the three Gunas in the human psychology. In the creation the three Gunas are all positive and important. See the chart below:

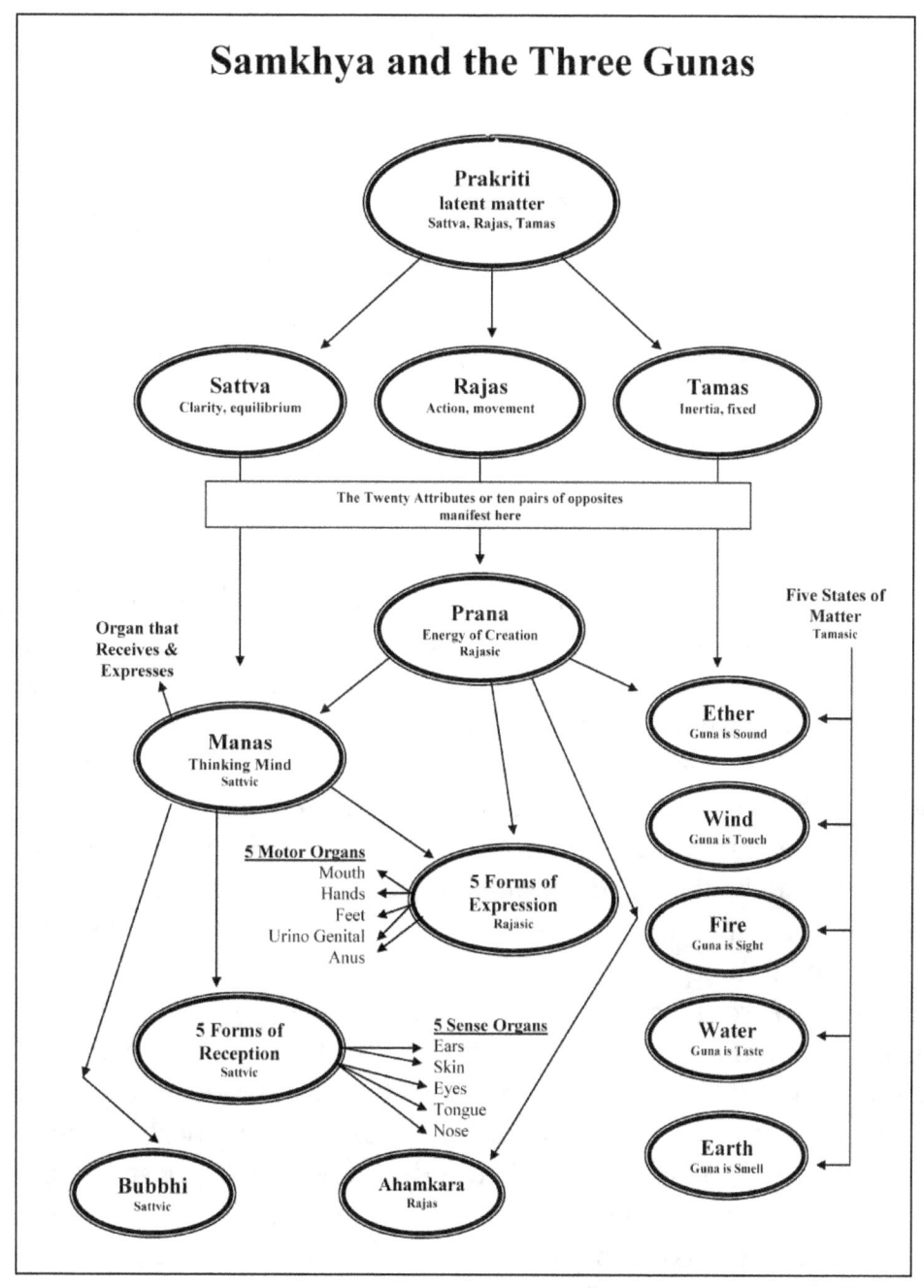

As we can see from the chart the three Gunas are the attributes of the cosmic Prakriti. Through Rajas the whole creation takes form. Under that creative action of Rajas, Sattva forms the mind and senses and Tamas the five elements. Thus, the creation is basically Rajasic in nature and needs all three Gunas in order to function correctly.

In terms of the human psychology Caraka points out that the rules are now different. The Gunas of rajas and Tamas are no-longer beneficial because the mind is the domain of Sattva – as seen in the chart. So Ayurvedic psychology sees the Gunas on a SUB LEVEL of the creation as indicated in the chart on page 3. Caraka also sees the mind as the realm of Sattva and the other two Gunas as causing problems.

Dosha vs. Guna

The issue of Prakriti is often confused between doshas and Gunas. The dosha are fixed at birth (conception) and do not change during life. The Gunas are different. They are modifiable right from birth and give us the freedom of "free will" that we humans prise above all else.

The amount of Sattva, rajas and Tamas that we demonstrate at birth depends on three factors:

1) Our vasanas that the Jivatman brings with it
2) The Guna dominance in our parents
3) Our early childhood environment

We can cultivate or develop the Gunas through effort and training. It is up to us what kind of Guna we choose to develop. If we do not make any effort to change our Guna dominance then we will adapt to our environment. This is known in Sanskrit as our associations. This demonstrates a law of nature: 'like increase like', and applies equally well to the psychology as it does in the physical domain. Hence, hanging out in a violent neighbourhood with drug dealers and murders will increase rajas and Tamas. In India the practice of Satsanga (sat = truth + sanga = association) exploits this mechanism of positive resonance. Unfortunately, the word satsang has now come to mean any idiot who sits on a platform and repeats spiritual words. Sat means "living in truth" in the Sattvic part of the mind – prior to conditioning.

You cannot change your basic metabolic nature (Prakriti). Does this mean that we are stuck mentally; condemned to the whims of our dominant mental dosha or doshas? Thankfully, the answer is no, we can cultivate the positive qualities of any of the three doshas, just as we can the three Gunas. Just as we can create a healthy functioning of Vata, Pitta and Kapha on a physiological level (healthy movement, digestion and cohesion), we can also cultivate the positive mental traits of the doshas. This is basically the fundament concept of Ayurvedic and Yogic psychology; development of Sattva in the mind increases the positive attributes of the three doshas.

This is where the three Gunas come into play, notably, the role of Sattva or equilibrium. Through conscious effort, we can cultivate the positive traits of the three doshas. The main thing to see here is that the contents of our minds are a choice – we can cultivate positive doshic traits of all the doshas – but this requires an effort on our part. If we fail to make any effort, we may succumb to the 'negative' traits of our doshas that form the foundation of the mental Prakriti. The methodology of this development is by using the three Gunas as a therapeutic tool.

Here is a review of the Gunas and their main qualities in the human mind:

Sattva gives: creativity, flexibility compassion, kindness, open, loving, caring, intelligent, humanitarian, development, direct

Rajas gives: dispersing, energetic, confused, indirect, aggressive, motivated, goal seeking, angry, controlling, manipulative, fanatical

Tamas: delusion, dullness, stupidity, blind spots, manipulating, violent, deceiving, dishonest, depression, degeneration, perverse

To be very clear **Rajas + Tamas** = violence and violent behaviour. Rajas alone is not "obscure" enough to hurt people or things and Tamas is not "active" enough to carry out harming other people. Hence, human society tends to be violent due the strong mixes of Rajas and Tamas.

Sattva	Rajas	Tamas
• Compassion • Flexable • Humanitarian • Responsive	• Dispersion • Energetic • Confused • Reactionary	• Blind spots • Stagnant • Delusion • Depression

In India there are different opinions about which Prakriti is Sattvic, Rajasic or Tamasic. In fact none of them are and all of them are. Any person can choose to become Rajasic, Tamasic or Sattvic according to their will and freedom of choice. As stated earlier the dominance of Gunas is determined by your parents and environment to a large extent – not your dosha dominance.

Hence, any doshic type can be more or less any Guna as illustrated in the chart below:

Mental Traits according to the Three Gunas			
	Vata	**Pitta**	**Kapha**
Sattvic	Intelligent, energetic, happy, adaptable, flexible, quick in communication, strong sense of human unity, enthusiastic, positive spirit, able to initiate things, loving, creative and movement orientated.	Intelligent, clear, happy, perceptive, discriminating, good will power, loving, clear communications, friendly, humanitarian, independent, dynamic, warm, courageous, sharing and teaching	Intelligent, calm, happy, peaceful, stable, consistent, loving, compassionate, forgiving, patient, devoted, receptive, nurturing, loyal, supportive, humanitarian, and faithful
Rajasic	Indecisive, unreliable, hyperactive, agitated, volatile, disturbed, distracted, nervous, anxious, overly talkative, superficial, noisy, disruptive, excitable, dispersed	Willful, impulsive, ambitious, aggressive, controlling, critical, dominating, reckless, manipulating, angry, proud, vain, frustrated, lustful	Controlling, attached, greedy, lustful, miserly, self-centered, materialistic, angry, proud, vain, overly sentimental, needing security, dominating
Tamasic	Depressed, fearful, servile, dishonest, secretive, destructive, self-destructive, drug addict, perverse, criminal, mentally disturbed, suicidal	Depressed, power hungry, dishonest, vile, vindictive, destructive, psychopath, criminal, dictator, drug dealer, drug addict, secretive, perverse, politician, criminal	Depressed, dishonest, dull, lethargic, slothful, apathetic, destructive, self-destructive, slow comprehension, misery, secretive, insensitive, drug addict, criminal, perverse

Basically the Guna dominance in the mind is called the content or "objects" of the mind. Caraka says in this sutra:

"*Mind transcends all sense perceptions. It is known as Sattva. Its action is determined by its contact with Jiva and* **the objects that reside in it (i.e., happiness, misery, etc.).** *Thus mind dictates all sense perceptions.*"
CS.SU.8.4

Therefore, what we hold in the mind is basically a reflection of the Guna dominance. For example, if I am depressed much of the time then it reflects a dominance of Tamas Guna. This tendency of depression mainly affects Kapha types, but this Tamas Guna can create depression in any type – Vata or Pitta – due to the lack of movement. So the chart above can be indicative and not final.

We will go into how the mind becomes conditioned in a future lesson on clinical psychology. For more information on this subject please consult my book *The Psychology of Transformation in Yoga* which gives a thorough discussion of the principle of Sattva, Rajas and Tamas in relation to psychology.

Conclusion

Mental Prakriti is pure by nature (Sattva) and is modified by Rajas and Tamas which make problems for the human psychology. Conditioned mind is the result of the Jiva, the parents and society that use Rajas and Tamas to "cover" the natural states of the mind. In the Ayurvedic analysis of mental Prakriti it is important to understand the basic conditioning of the patient (culture, religion, etc.) because this establishes the doshic orientation of the mind. In other words, the Gunas (conditioning) give their qualities to the dosha Prakriti in the mind; e.g. Vata-Sattva, Vata-Rajas or Vata-Tamas.

This understanding is needed to help a patient overcome problems and to determine which therapies they will be able to carry out on their own at home. Remember that all of us are basically dominated by Rajas and Tamas and through our own effort we increase Sattva to be able to reduce and balance out the difficult aspects of the other two Gunas.

Here is a Prakriti evaluation form that can be used alone or in conjunction with the questionnaire. It is suggested to do ten evaluations with either patients or friends in order to become familiar with the concepts presented in the last four chapters. Unless these ideas are put into practice they will remain an intellectual concept. This may lead to a superficial judgment of Prakriti evaluations.

PRAKRITI EVALUATION
CASE STUDY TEMPLATE

VITAL STATISTICS
NAME:
ADDRESS:
AGE:
SEX:
PROFESSION:

For each category below, note your observations (20 Gunas, qualities, etc.) then your conclusion about the dominant dosha(s). Refer to Chapters 10 & 11 for guidance:

PART 1 - PHYSICAL & METABOLIC EVALUATION
FACE & HEAD
TONGUE
HANDS, NAILS & WRISTS
OTHER PHYSICAL TRAITS (Example: bone thickness, skin, hair, etc.)
APPETITE (AGNI)
DIGESTION (AGNI)

ELIMINATION
CIRCULATION
MENSTRUATION
OTHER METABOLIC TRAITS
RESPONSE TO ENVIRONMENT
RESISTANCE TO DISEASE (IMMUNITY)
DISEASE TENDENCIES
OTHER GENERAL OBSERVATIONS
TOTALS (PHYSICAL ASPECTS)

Now evaluate some of the following mental aspects – note down both dosha and Maha Guna for each category to determine the mental Prakriti (refer to Chapters 12 & 13 for guidance):

PART 2 - PSYCHOLOGICAL EVALUATION (USE BOTH DOSHA AND MAHA GUNA)
MENTAL CLARITY
MENTAL STABILITY
SPEECH HABITS
PERSONAL RELATIONSHIP TENDENCIES
EMOTIONAL TENDENCIES

NEUROTIC TENDENCIES
FAITH IN LIFE
MEMORY
DREAM TENDENCIES
SLEEP TENDENCIES
LIFE GOALS
MATERIAL VALUES
WORK HABITS
EATING HABITS
GENERAL HABITS
RELATIONSHIP TO MONEY
SPENDING HABITS
FRIENDSHIPS
SOCIAL RELATIONS
GENERAL MENTAL NATURE
ANY OTHER PSYCHOLOGICAL TRAITS (list)
TOTAL (MENTAL ASPECTS)

Note here your thoughts about the overall Prakriti taking into account the information from Chapters 10, 11, 12 and 13. This is the place to make a synthesis of all information and try to come up with a working hypothesis of Prakriti for the person.

PART 3 - OVERALL CONCLUSIONS & DISCUSSION

Study Questions for Chapter Thirteen

1. Why is the mind healthy by nature?

2. What does the functional aspect of the mind relate to?

3. The Sanskrit word "Manas" can have two meanings; what are they?

4. Why do we need to determine the Guna dominance when doing Prakriti analysis?

5. Why do normal people tend to be dominate in Rajas and Tamas?

6. The dosha are fixed at birth and do not change during life. Why are the Gunas different.?

7. The amount of Sattva, Rajas and Tamas that we demonstrate at birth depends on which three factors?

8. What are the main qualities of Sattva in the human mind?

9. What are the main qualities of Rajas in the human mind?

10. What are the main qualities of Tamas in the human mind?

GLOSSARY

Agni: first of three cosmic principals; god of fire; digestive fire

Agnivasa: the sage who first complied the text now known as the Caraka Samhita

Allopathy: western medicine, modern medicine

Apana vayu: one of the five pranas; the prana that controls all evacuation, called the downward breath; resides in the lower abdomen; one of the five forms of Vata Dosha

Aphrodisiac: any substance that promotes health to the reproductive organs

Astanga Hrdayam: one of the three ancient Ayurvedic texts of medicine

Atma: pure consciousness; Brahman

Atreya: the teacher of Agnivasa and source of the Caraka Samhita

Ayurveda: the part of the Vedas dealing with health; the science of life: longevity

Brahma: consciousness or God in an absolute sense; one of the three aspects of God, the creator, or creative aspect; the founder of Ayurveda

Brahmin: the learned class of people in Vedic society; priests

Bramhacharya: abidance in Brahma or God

Caraka Samhita: the oldest surviving text of Ayurveda

Chit: consciousness

Consciousness: as used in this book, the Substratum or Source of all manifestation

Constitution: an individual's unique mix of the three Doshas.

Dosha: Sanskrit for humor; lit: "that which stains"

Dhatu: tissue; there are seven different tissue levels in Ayurveda (rasa, Rakta, mamsa, meda, asthi, Majja, shukra) - plasma, blood, muscle, fat, bone, bone marrow and nerve tissue, and reproductive fluids

Energetic Impressions: in Sanskrit there are two kinds: Vasanas & Samskaras, these are latent, unconscious or stored impressions and current mental impressions; these impressions are stored in the subtle body; Yoga says that these impressions are what cause us to incarnate in another life, unless they are allowed to surface to consciousness; these impressions along with prana create what we call mind.

Five elements: see Five States of Matter

Five States of Matter: commonly called the Five Elements; the five states of material are: mass, liquidity, transformation, movement, and the field in which they function; also called: ether, air, fire, water & earth

Guna: quality or attribute; there are three Maha Gunas: Sattva, Rajas, and Tamas; and there are twenty Gurvadi Gunas

197

Kapha: one of the three humors; controls water and earth elements.

Karma: action; the cosmic law of for every action there is a reaction

Latent impression: see Energetic impressions.

Marma: the acupressure and acupuncture points of Ayurveda.

Maya: the illusion that every exists as separate from God

Mind: thoughts moving through consciousness, giving the illusion of continuity; the combination of prana and vasanas; Manas

Ojas: there are two kinds, 1) the essence of food metabolized by the seen Dhatus; 2) humans are born with eight drops of Ojas in the heart; together they form the basis of basic vitality and the immune system by storing Prana; it is reputed to be white or golden in color

Pitta: one of the three humors; controls fire and water elements.

Prakriti: the dynamic energy of consciousness; natal constitution; nature

Prana: pra = before, ana = breath; the vital force; it arises from substratum of pure consciousness with intelligence, Agni, and love, together they create the individualized consciousness. There are five major pranas in the human body, prana, apana, samana, udana and vyana, they arise from the cosmic prana

Prana vayu: chief of the five pranas in the body, called the outward going breath, it resides in the head and the heart; one of the five forms of Vata Dosha

Pranayama: awareness of breath; method of breath observation used to regulate the mind, thereby the physical and mental health

Purusha: the inert aspect of consciousness; Sat Chit Ananda

Rajas: one of the three Gunas; action, movement, bright, energy, aggression, aggravated mind, achievement, and strong emotions.

Rasa: lit. taste, juice; first Dhatu

Samana vayu: one of the five pranas in the body; called the equalizing prana it resides in the navel region; one of the five forms of Vata Dosha

Samsara: the concept that we are separate from God; suffering; illusion.

Samskaras: Innate energetic impressions, see *energetic impressions*.

Sattva: one of the three Gunas; purity, peace, calm, beauty, happiness, quite obedient mind, and stable emotions.

Srotas: channels in the Ayurvedic system

Substratum: equal to: The Absolute, Consciousness, God, Love, Brahman, Atman, Self or Source.

Sushruta Samhita: one of the three ancient Ayurvedic texts of medicine

Tamas: one of the three Gunas; inertia, dull, depressed, void, stupid, lazy, despair, and self-destructive emotions.

Udana vayu: one of the five pranas in the body; called the upward moving breath, it is seated in the throat; one of the five forms of Vata Dosha

Vikriti: lit. that which covers Prakriti; pathology

Vasanas: Latent energetic impression, see energetic impressions.

Vata: that which moves; one of the three Dosha; controls wind (air) and ether elements.

Vayu: the God of the Wind; another name for Vata; another name for prana.

Vedas: Literally it means knowledge, but used here to mean the Book of Knowledge, the oldest book in the world; there are four Vedas.

Vyana vayu: one of the five pranas in the body; called the equalizing breath it unifies all the other pranas and the body, it is defused throughout the body; one of the five forms of Vata Dosha

Yoga: Union; methodology that which leads one back to the original Source; generally understood to mean a path or a practice leading to the Divine.

BIBLIOGRAPHY

Bibliography of Classical Texts

Astanga Hrdayam, vols; I - III, trans. Murthy, Prof. K.R. Srikantha, Varanasi, India; Krishnadas Academy, 3rd ed. 1996

Astanga Samgraha, vols; I - III, trans. Murthy, Prof. K.R. Srikantha, Varanasi, India; Chaukhamba Orientalia, 8th ed. 2004

Bhāvaprakāśā, vols; I - II, trans. Murthy, Prof. K.R. Srikantha, Varanasi, India; Krishnadas Academy, 1998

Caraka Samhitā, vols; I - VII, trans. Dash, Vaidya Bhagwan & Sharma, Dr. R.K., Varanasi, India; Chowkhamba Series Office, 1992-2002.

Caraka Samhitā, vols; I - IV, trans. Sharma, Prof. P.V., Varanasi, India; Chowkhamba, 1987-2002.

Madhava Nidanam, trans. Murthy, Prof. K.R. Srikantha, Varanasi, India; Chaukhamba Orientalia, 4th ed. 2004

Suśruta Samhitā, vols; I - III, trans. K.K. Bhishagratna, Varanasi, India; Chaukhamba Sanskrit Pratishthan, 1998- 2002

INDEX

ABOUT THE AUTHOR

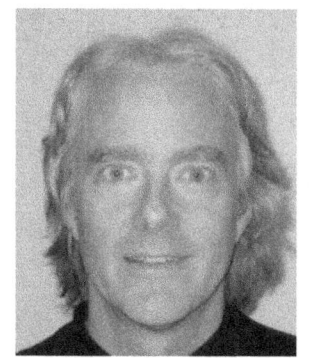 Vaidya Atreya Smith is the author of six books published in nine different languages on the art of Indian medicine and healing. Since 1998 he directs the European Institute of Vedic Studies, Switzerland. Since 1987 he has studied with a number of Indian professors of Ayurveda in India. He continues his studies on Ayurveda with his teachers in India. He has a BSc in Biology and in 2005 was awarded the title of Vaidya in Varanasi for his work in Ayurveda. From 1987 Atreya has been a professional in health care working with thousands of patients in countries all over the world. He is a professional herbalist and the member of several professional organizations. Atreya has written courses on Ayurvedic nutrition and Dravyaguna for Westerners and is one of the most sought after teachers of Ayurveda in Europe. Atreya and his Institute are affiliated with a number of universities and institutes throughout the world for the promotion of Ayurveda and other Indian sciences.

Vaidya Atreya Smith offers a three level training program to anyone who is interested in learning Ayurveda. The first part of the program is offered by Vaidya Atreya Smith using the latest technology - advanced learning methods on an E-learning platform. This program lasts one school year. After completion of the first part (e-learning) students qualify for the second level - a three week clinical studies program with Dr. Sunil V. Joshi, in Nagpur, India. The third level is on Dravyaguna for Westerners and is taught by Atreya through e-learning. This program also lasts one school year. For students who diplomas from other schools it is possible to join our program in India or on medicinal plants. For further information look at our websites.

www.atreya.com
www.ayurvedicnutrition.com

To insure the preservation of medicinal plants around the world Vaidya Atreya Smith has started several projects to actively protect this important natural resource. Information on the vision and how to support it can be found on this website:

www.eivs.org